Athletic Training
Student Guide
to Success

Athletic Training Student Guide to Success

Lynn Van Ost, MEd, RN, PT, ATC
Sports Physical Therapy Institute, PA
Princeton, New Jersey

Karen Manfré, MA, ATR
Head Athletic Trainer
Hunterton Central Regional High School
Flemington, New Jersey

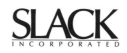

SLACK
INCORPORATED

6900 Grove Road, Thorofare, NJ 08086

141100

Publisher: John H. Bond
Editorial Director: Amy E. Drummond

The material in this book has been compiled to help the student review and prepare for the certification exam. The author and the publisher are not responsible for errors or omissions, or for consequences from application of the book and makes no warranty, expressed or implied, in regard to the contents of the book.

The work SLACK Incorporated publishes is peer-reviewed. Prior to publication, recognized leaders in the field, educators, and clinicians provide important feedback on the concepts and content that we publish. We welcome feedback on this work.

Van Ost, Lynn.
      Athletic training student guide to success / Lynn Van Ost, Karen Manfré.
         p. cm.
      Includes bibliographical references.
      ISBN 1-55642-379-9 (alk. paper)
         1. Athletic trainers. I. Manfré, Karen, 1952- II. Title.

RC1210 .V36 2000
617.1'027--dc21   00-030069

Printed in the United States of America.
Published by: SLACK Incorporated
                     6900 Grove Road
                     Thorofare, NJ 08086-9447 USA
                     Telephone: 856-848-1000
                     Fax: 856-853-5991
                     www.slackbooks.com

Contact SLACK Incorporated for more information about other books in this field or about the availability of our books from distributors outside the United States.

Last digit is print number: 10 9 8 7 6 5 4 3 2 1

To our families and special friends
(you know who you are)
who have taught us the true meaning of perseverance.
Thank you for all your support and patience with our endless projects.
At least this one is done!

Contents

Dedication . . . .*v*

Acknowledgments . . . .*ix*

About the Authors . . . .*xi*

Introduction . . . .*xiii*

Chapter I: Study Techniques and Test-Taking Strategies 1
      Improving Concentration *1*
      Additional Study Suggestions *2*
      Time Management *3*
      Specific Test-Taking Strategies *4*
      Decreasing Your Test Anxiety *4*
      What to Bring to the Examination *5*

Chapter II: General Information and the Examination Format 7
      Eligibility and Applying for the NATA Certification Examination *7*
      Development of the NATABOC Certification Examination *9*
      The NATABOC Certification Examination Format *10*

Chapter III: Written Examination Sample Questions 13
      Athletic Training Domains
      Prevention of Athletic Injury and Illness *13*
      Recognition, Evaluation, and Immediate Care of Injuries *24*
      Rehabilitation of Athletic Injuries *41*
      Health Care Administration *57*
      Professional Development and Responsibility *63*

      Core Subject Areas
      Athletic Training Evaluation *71*
      Human Anatomy *78*
      Human Physiology *85*
      Exercise Physiology *90*
      Biomechanics *95*
      Psychology *99*
      Nutrition *104*
      Pharmacology *107*
      Physics *109*
      Administration *112*

Chapter IV: Written Simulation Sample Questions 115
      Problem I *116*
      Problem II *118*
      Problem III *119*
      Problem IV *120*
      Problem V *121*
      Problem VI *123*
      Problem VII *124*
      Problem VIII *125*
      Problem IX *126*
      Problem X *127*
      Problem XI *128*
      Problem XII *129*
      Problem XIII *131*
      Problem XIV *132*
      Problem XV *134*
      Problem XVI *136*
      Problem XVII *136*
      Problem XVIII *138*
      Problem XIX *139*
      Problem XX *140*

Chapter V: Practical Practice Sample Questions 143
      Problem I *143*
      Problem II *144*
      Problem III *144*
      Problem IV *145*

Problem V *145*
Problem VI *146*
Problem VII *147*
Problem VIII *147*
Problem IX *148*
Problem X *148*
Problem XI *148*
Problem XII *149*
Problem XIII *149*
Problem XIV *150*
Problem XV *150*
Problem XVI *150*
Problem XVII *151*
Problem XVIII *152*
Problem XIX *152*
Problem XX *153*

Chapter VI: What to Do if You Do Not Pass the First Time .... .155

Appendix A: Sample Study Calendar and Daily Log .... .157

Appendix B: Answer Key—Written Examination Sample Questions .... .159
                   Athletic Training Domains
                   Prevention of Athletic Injury and Illness .... .159
                   Recognition, Evaluation, and Immediate Care of Injuries .... .162
                   Rehabilitation of Athletic Injuries .... .169
                   Health Care Administration .... .174
                   Professional Development and Responsibility .... .176
                   Core Subject Areas
                   Athletic Training Evaluation .... .178
                   Human Anatomy .... .181
                   Human Physiology .... .183
                   Exercise Physiology .... .184
                   Biomechanics .... .186
                   Psychology .... .187
                   Nutrition .... .188
                   Pharmacology .... .189
                   Physics .... .190
                   Administration .... .191

Appendix C: Answer Key—Written Simulation Sample Questions .... .193
                   Problem I .... .193
                   Problem II .... .197
                   Problem III .... .199
                   Problem IV .... .201
                   Problem V .... .203
                   Problem VI .... .205
                   Problem VII .... .207
                   Problem VIII .... .208
                   Problem IX .... .210
                   Problem X .... .211
                   Problem XI .... .213
                   Problem XII .... .215
                   Problem XIII .... .217
                   Problem XIV .... .219
                   Problem XV .... .224
                   Problem XVI .... .227
                   Problem XVII .... .228
                   Problem XVIII .... .231
                   Problem XIX .... .233
                   Problem XX .... .234

Bibliography .... .239

Acknowledgments

We would like to extend a sincere thank you to many individuals who have helped us along the way in completing this book. First and foremost, we would like to thank Amy Drummond and SLACK Incorporated for being so enthusiastic and supportive during our journey through the jungle of publication. Certainly a huge thank you is extended to Ann Louise Smith, Judd E. Strauss, and Peggy Bardes for the endless hours of typing and editing; this book could not have been produced without you.

Lynn Van Ost graduated in 1982 with a BS in nursing from West Chester State College, West Chester, PA, in 1987 from Temple University, Philadelphia, PA, with a Master's in sports medicine/athletic training, and in 1988 from Temple University with a second Bachelor's in physical therapy. In addition to treating the general orthopedic population as a physical therapist, she has worked with both amateur and professional athletes and has over 11 years' experience as an athletic trainer working with Olympic level elite athletes at numerous international events, including the 1992 and 1996 Summer Olympic games. She currently works in a physical therapy private practice and occasionally serves as a volunteer athletic trainer for US Field Hockey.

Karen Manfré graduated from SUNY College at Brockport in 1977 with a BS in physical education/athletic training and from Rider University with a Master's in educational administration in 1999. She has been in education for over 20 years and has worked as an athletic trainer at many levels of competition including professional, elite, and intercollegiate. She currently serves as the head athletic trainer for Hunterdon Central Regional High School in Flemington, NJ.

Introduction

This study guide for the NATA Board of Certification (NATABOC) certification examination was inspired and developed as a result of a strong passion for our profession. Athletic training is a unique health care profession in that the athletic trainer is often in the position of experiencing the results of his or her efforts. The athletes' wins are our wins; their losses our losses. We become a friend, mentor, counselor, teacher, guardian, protector, and healer. It takes a special individual to become a proficient and dedicated professional athletic trainer. Long hours are spent in the training room, classroom, and on courts and fields preparing for the final examination that will allow you to place the letters ATC behind your name.

Our intent in writing this study guide is to assist you in accomplishing that final goal of passing the NATABOC Entry-Level Athletic Training examination. It is an accumulation of dedicated research and past experience. We have included a section on study techniques to assist you in your preparation for the examination, and a general overview of the examination format to help you organize your thoughts.

This guide has been divided into six major areas: study techniques, general information and the examination format, sample written questions, sample written simulation questions, sample questions for the practical examination, and practical tips and advice for those who do not pass the first time.

The written questions have been organized according to the core subject areas of athletic training and NATA Education Task Force educational domains to allow you to assess subjects you may be weak in, and where your strengths lie. Although this study guide will assist you in preparing for the certification examination, it should not be used in place of your textbooks or other sources of study from your school curriculum. It is not intended to be a "practice" examination; it is meant only to be used as an adjunct source of information and to tie together everything you have learned in the classroom and during your fieldwork.

In Chapters I and II, "Study Techniques and Test-Taking Strategies" and "General Information and the Examination Format," we have provided some specific tools to assist you in organizing yourself up to 6 months prior to the examination. Chapter III consists of 725 study questions. Four hundred of the questions are a "mixed bag" of subjects derived from the NATA Education Task Force athletic training educational domains. The final 325 questions cover most of the core subject areas of athletic training. Chapter IV includes 20 written simulation problems, testing your ability to make appropriate judgment calls and improve your problem-solving skills. Each problem presents a specific scenario with several possible options that you can choose to follow. Chapter V is a simulation for the practical examination. This section is comprised of 20 problems that are designed to test your manual athletic training skills.

The final chapter is directed at helping you if your test results are not favorable. We have included some suggestions on how to deal with the immediate difficulties not passing may cause, and how to begin the process of developing a new approach for your next attempt. Provided you have applied the information you have learned in the classroom and on the field to the study strategies we have offered in this manual, you will not need to read this final chapter. We wish you luck and look forward to welcoming you as a colleague.

Chapter 1

STUDY TECHNIQUES AND TEST-TAKING STRATEGIES

The most obvious question that comes to mind when preparing for the NATA Board of Certification athletic trainer certification exam is "Where do I start?" Just the thought of studying for this examination can be overwhelming. There seems to be so much information and so little time to absorb it all. The good news is that none of this information should be new to you, so consider this a review of what you already know.

The best way to prevent you from feeling overwhelmed and to develop the motivation to study is to begin by taking small steps toward your goal. The first step is to learn new study strategies or improve the ones you currently find effective. Learning how to concentrate and organize your time in an efficient manner is the basis of good study skills. Remember, it is not necessarily the quantity of time you spend but the quality of time that counts.

IMPROVING CONCENTRATION

Concentration may be defined as the ability to focus on the task at hand. Here are some suggestions to improve your ability to concentrate while studying.

Eliminate Environmental Distractions

- Select one or two special study areas, preferably a place that is quiet and secluded.
- Agree with those with whom you live (eg, roommates, spouses/relatives, and children) on a time you will be free to socialize.
- Hang a "Do Not Disturb" sign on your door, wear a specific item of clothing, or tie a brightly colored ribbon to the door as your signal to others that you do not wish to be interrupted.
- Inform those who find it necessary to interrupt you during your study time on a regular basis that it is important they do not talk to you until you are ready to do so. Make sure you send a clear but tactful message, as they might not be aware that they are interfering with your ability to concentrate.
- Ignore distracting sights and sounds such as the telephone, television, or loud music. Although some students state that they study better with music in the background, a silent room will provide no distractions at all. It is best to use your answering machine or voice mail so you are not tempted to answer the phone.

Reduce Mind Wandering

- Stand up and walk away from your material when you find yourself wandering. Then come back and try again.
- Concentrate only on the material you are reviewing. If you have errands or something suddenly pops into your mind, write it down on a note pad and tackle it at a later time.

- Make sure you stay in good shape, both physically and mentally. It is important to eat, sleep, and exercise routinely. You cannot concentrate or perform adequately if you are hungry or are a victim of sleep deprivation. Get out and exercise; it will relax you and clear your mind.

- If you have other major concerns you are currently worrying about, such as personal problems at home or at work, make sure you attend to them when you are not studying. Try to find a way to resolve the problems as soon as possible so they do not distract you from the goal at hand.

- Remember to reward your studying with a social event or some quiet time alone doing an enjoyable activity that requires little focused concentration. Set a goal for your reward, such as reviewing a particular subject completely and to your satisfaction. Be careful not to set up your "time off" as your goal.

Improve Your Concentration

- Develop a good attitude toward the subject you are studying. Have an inquisitive mind; ask yourself additional questions and search your books and notes for the answers. Skim through the textbook before reviewing a subject or create games for yourself. Try to make your study time as exciting and challenging as you can. The power of positive thinking will help you ride the tide.

- Break down major areas into smaller components for study (eg, instead of tackling anatomy, try a smaller subject like the muscles of the lower extremity).

- When you get tired, take a break. Get something to drink or eat or take a stroll around the neighborhood. Try to become more aware of the amount of time you are able to adequately concentrate. It is probably best to study for only 2 to 3 hours at a time before taking a 10-minute break.

- Make sure you do not vary your study spots. The areas you have chosen for studying should be utilized only to study. Try to select a specific time to study and do not get involved in any other activity in that area once you are through. Being consistent with both the time and place you choose to study will train you to be more efficient.

ADDITIONAL STUDY SUGGESTIONS

- **Form or attend a study group.** Make sure the individuals you ask to join the group are eager learners and are willing to participate on a regular basis. This will assure everyone that each person is contributing his or her fair share of work. Make sure the goals of the group are clearly defined so time is not wasted, and that everyone has an equal role in accomplishing those goals.

- **Textbook review.** Only refer to your textbooks when it is necessary to review areas on which you are weak or to study a topic in more detail. To try to read any of your textbooks from beginning to end is completely ineffective and will only cause you to panic.

- **Examination review courses.** Some schools will offer review courses for the examination. These courses are often given in the summer when the school curriculum is less intense. It might be wise to contact a school that offers an NATA-accredited curriculum to see if a review course is offered.

- **Class notes.** Your notes from your classes should comprise the majority of your study materials. The subjects outlined by the NATABOC as requirements for candidates planning to take the certification examination should have been sufficiently covered in your curriculum. If you are unsure of anything that was covered in a particular class, contact the professor so that he or she might help you clear up your questions.

- **Audiovisual aids.** Audiovisual aids may help to clarify a confusing topic. It sometimes helps to be able to see or hear how a task is performed and have the ability to rerun the task several times to fully understand how it is done. If you learn better by hearing and seeing, ask your instructor or supervisor where you might obtain tapes or instructional videos (eg, handling an unconscious athlete, strength training techniques, etc).

- **Practice with a buddy.** If you find you do not work well in groups but need to practice specific skills, enlist the assistance of a friend, especially another candidate whose needs are similar to yours. Feedback is important for accuracy and timing, and only someone familiar with what you are trying to accomplish can give you helpful insight. Working with someone in the same boat can also help alleviate your anxieties. The athletic trainer who is endorsing you should also be available to help you practice a skill that may be particularly weak.
- **Flash cards.** Make up flash cards with questions and answers and carry them with you. This technique works especially well when studying factual information such as anatomy, kinesiology, or therapeutic modalities. They are easy to carry and allow you to study in bits and pieces anytime, anywhere.

TIME MANAGEMENT

It is essential that you learn to organize your time and develop some specific test-taking techniques. Careful planning of your time will allow you to work more efficiently. Developing a purposeful calendar of events will allow you to prioritize your tasks and accomplish them step by step. Preparation is the key to success. Time spent organizing and planning in advance will reduce your anxiety and allow you to think straight under pressure. The following ideas might be of help if you find either one or both of the above mentioned areas to be a source of frustration.

- Plan a schedule for studying by creating a chart dividing the months into weeks and weeks into days and hours (see Appendix A).
- Fill in this chart with your planned study times, activities, and "down time." Keep a record of your study pattern and review it on a weekly basis. If you are not spending enough time studying, where are you spending the time?
- When scheduling study times, be sure to allow yourself additional time for your harder topics. This will help you to avoid cramming, which is ineffective.
- Concentrate your study efforts on clinical situations, diseases, or areas with which you are not as familiar. For example, if you have never dealt with an athlete with a thoracic injury or a life-threatening allergic reaction, focus a bit more of your attention on those topics. Get more information until you are satisfied that the topic is well covered.
- Know the date of your examination and make sure all the preliminaries are taken care of ahead of time (eg, your application materials are in, your CPR card is current, etc). This will help you organize your calendar.
- Think about the following questions and answer them to identify how you manage your time:

  When are you most alert? In the morning, afternoon, or evening? What time is optimal for you to study?

  How much sleep do you require to be most alert and able to concentrate?

  When do you prefer to have your meals?

  How much time do you like to exercise? What time is optimal for exercising?

  How much time do you allow for relaxation or fun activities when you study?

  What other priorities do you have in your life and when are the best times to address them?

SPECIFIC TEST-TAKING STRATEGIES

By following a few simple guidelines when you actually sit down to take the test, you may eliminate a number of silly mistakes that can easily be made as a result of being too anxious.

- If you think of any information you are afraid you might forget, write it down on the back of the exam.
- Preview your test and look over the types and number of questions given.
- Read all the test instructions thoroughly before starting.
- Budget your time; note how many questions you must answer for each section and how much each question is worth. Estimate how much time you have to answer each question.
- If you are unsure of something on the examination, be sure to ask the proctor to explain it. Do not be afraid to inquire!
- Make sure you read the entire question and all the answers to the question before deciding which choice is best.
- Answer the easiest questions first. If you are unsure of an answer, go with your first choice.
- If you cannot decide on the best answer to a question, place a check or question mark in the margin and come back to it later.
- Keep track of your time during the examination with your watch or a wall clock.
- Rephrase difficult questions in your own words, but be sure not to change the meaning of the question.
- For the written examination only (not the written simulation), answer all the questions even if you have to guess. Do not leave any question unanswered.
- Once you are finished, check your answers carefully to make sure you have not made any careless mistakes. One skipped question or mismarked answer can throw off the rest of your answers.
- For multiple choice questions, if you have a question that has "all of the above" or "none of the above" as possible answers, go through each of the other answers and place a true or false next to it. If all or none of the answers are true or false, then all or none of the above applies.

DECREASING YOUR TEST ANXIETY

Everyone feels some level of anxiety before taking a test; it is a normal response to feeling challenged. However, it is important to take control of your feelings so they do not overwhelm you and paralyze your thought process. Here are some ideas that you might try to make you more comfortable.

- Prepare early, approximately 6 months prior to the exam. Check to make sure you have everything in order to apply to take the test. If you are well prepared before the actual examination, it will be one less thing to worry about. Assuming you have met all the requirements, this is the time to start organizing your study plan.
- Know the location of the test site and leave enough time to get there early. Make sure to check the weather reports the night before to allow any changes in planning. If you live a good distance away, stay at a hotel the night before.
- Try to relax the night before the examination. Go out to dinner or take in a fun movie with friends. This will help you to sleep well the night prior to the examination. Just be sure not to stay up late! You will want to be very alert the next morning.
- Eat a good breakfast the morning of the examination. You will not be able to concentrate if you are hungry, and you need fuel to stay alert.

- Make sure to dress comfortably. Wear clothing that is loose, such as a neat sweatsuit (without your school logo), or layers of clothing so you can make adjustments if the room temperature is not to your liking. It is best to appear professional. Do not wear a hat or bandana on your head, as this may attract attention.

- Do not cram the morning of the examination; this will only stress you out. It might help to scan through one or two small topics prior to the test, but in general, you will know all you are going to know by that time anyway.

- While waiting for the test, try stretching a bit or run in place. If you know how to do progressive relaxation (ie, progressively tensing and relaxing your muscles from head to toe), feel free to try it. Locate the bathroom and water fountain so you know where they are.

- Close your eyes and take some deep breaths; try to think positively and confidently. Remember, you have prepared yourself for this! If you go blank or find yourself panicking during the test, put your pencil down, close your eyes, and take a deep breath. Count to 10 or until you can focus again.

- Do not rehash your performance after the examination. What is done is done. Try to forget it for a couple of days. Plan to do something fun and stress-free after it is over.

- Do not compare yourself to your friends. You did the best you could and every candidate's test scores will vary. Do not allow your score to be a measure of your self-worth.

WHAT TO BRING TO THE EXAMINATION

Be sure to bring the following items with you on the day of the examination:
- A map to the test site with written directions.
- Telephone numbers for the test site and NATABOC.
- Your test admission ticket.
- A photo ID.
- Your confirmation notice from the NATABOC.
  Change for a pay phone, if necessary.
- A watch.
- Two or three #2 pencils.
- A clean eraser.
- Tissues.
- Reading glasses if necessary.
- Money for lunch.
- Proof of change of address or name change, if applicable.

Chapter II

GENERAL INFORMATION AND THE EXAMINATION FORMAT

ELIGIBILITY AND APPLYING FOR THE NATIONAL ATHLETIC TRAINERS' ASSOCIATION CERTIFICATION EXAMINATION

The National Athletic Trainer's Association Professional Education Committee (NATA-PEC) was originally formed by the NATABOC to monitor the curriculum and field experiences provided by those schools offering athletic training programs. It was this committee's responsibility to ensure that all programs designed to prepare students to become certified athletic trainers met and maintained the academic and clinical standards set by the NATABOC. At the time of this manual's printing, the NATA-PEC had since been replaced by the NATA Education Council (NATA-EC). This council is charged with setting the guidelines for the academic and clinical education of those students enrolled in accredited athletic training education programs.

Since it is not within the scope of this manual to include all the current policy changes being made by the NATA-EC regarding athletic training education, nor is it the intent of the authors to have this manual be used as a complete source of these changes, it is best to obtain information pertaining to these developments directly from the NATA-EC if you have specific questions or concerns.

Presently, those candidates who are eligible to take the NATA certification examination must have completed a program of study in athletic training that has been accredited by the Commission on Accreditation of Allied Health Education Programs (CAAHEP) or a program of study that follows the current internship route.

Those candidates who have entered an accredited athletic training curriculum must have successfully completed the athletic training program in no less than 2 academic years and must have received their bachelor's degree from the college or university at which they completed their coursework. Athletic training hours that have been accumulated more than 5 years from the application date are not accepted by the NATABOC. A candidate may also take the examination the second semester of his or her senior year provided all the prerequisites have been met and the endorsing athletic trainer has confirmed this in writing.

A CAAHEP-accredited athletic training program is divided into two components: clinical education and field experience. The clinical education component incorporates academic courses or academic credit that meets the requirements of the Joint Review Committee—Athletic Training (JRC-AT) guidelines. These courses are designed to teach the student athletic trainer the clinical skills of the profession and provide a venue in which he or she may practice those skills. It has been recommended by the NATA-EC that these courses provide an academic syllabi and/or a clinical instruction manual that outlines the educational objectives and clinical skill outcomes. These outcomes are derived from the *Entry-Level Athletic Training Clinical Proficiencies*. The individual university or college determines the amount of academic credit assigned to a given course according to the institution's individual guidelines. Clinical academic coursework may include an internship or externship or clinical laboratory class in addition to, but not in lieu of, formal academic clinical courses. Students are assigned to a designated approved clinical instructor (ACI) who is responsible for on-site daily supervision and the evaluation of the student's global performance.

The accredited athletic training program also includes 800 hours of athletic training experience, which must be performed under the supervision of a NATABOC certified athletic trainer. The majority of these hours must be fulfilled in the primary setting (ie, athletic training room) in which the minimum hours of direct supervision by an ATC are accumulated. The athletic training room must be located within an educational institution or professional sports venue and provides comprehensive athletic health care services (such as pre-practice and pre-game preparation, emergency and rehabilitative services, etc.) to a competitive athletic population. Approved field experience hours may also be accumulated at a secondary setting such as an on-campus satellite athletic training room and during athletic practices and events (on and off campus). Other clinical sites, such as a sportsmedicine center or emergency room, may be incorporated as adjunct affiliations.

At the time of this book's publication, the internship route to certification still exists and must be addressed. It is important to mention, however, that as of January 1, 2004, the NATABOC will be eliminating this program. The candidate who desires to meet the NATABOC requirements for certification as an intern must do so prior to December 31, 2003.

As with the candidates who have entered an accredited academic curriculum program, the internship candidate must fulfill both requirements for NATABOC-approved formal coursework and field experiences. The internship candidate must also complete his or her athletic training program over a period of at least 2 academic years, and any field experience hours that are accumulated more than 5 years from the application date are considered unacceptable by the NATABOC.

Unlike the accredited curriculum candidate, the internship candidate must submit to the NATABOC an official transcript that verifies the student has completed at least one formal core course in each of the following seven areas of study: health, human anatomy, kinesiology/biomechanics, human physiology, exercise physiology, and basic and advanced athletic training. A course on therapeutic modalities and rehabilitation (as separate entities) are the only courses that may serve to substitute for an advanced athletic training course. The basic and athletic training courses may not be taken outside of the United States unless the instructor in a foreign university is NATABOC certified. As of January 1, 2000, both the basic and advanced athletic training courses must include information pertaining to the prevention of athletic injuries, recognition and treatment of acute athletic injuries, evaluation of athletic injuries, therapeutic modalities, and the rehabilitation of athletic injuries.

The field experience for the internship candidate differs from the accredited athletic training program in that the internship candidate must complete 1500 hours of hands-on experience under the direct supervision of an NATABOC-certified athletic trainer. Five hundred of the required 1500 hours may be obtained at an adjunct clinical setting such as a sportsmedicine center, sports camp, or under the direct supervision of an athletic trainer certified by the Canadian Athletic Therapist's Association. The remaining 1000 hours must be acquired in an athletic training room setting in a secondary school, intercollegiate setting, or with a professional sports team. A Verification of Hours Form must be filled out by each certified trainer who has supervised acceptable fieldwork hours. These verification forms must be submitted with the certification examination application when the field experience is completed.

In general, hours that are supervised by anyone other than an NATABOC-certified athletic trainer, hours traveling to away games, and hours accumulated 5 years prior to the date of application for the certification examination will not be accepted by the NATABOC. In addition, any field experience hours that have been supervised by an athletic trainer who is a candidate's employer, family member, or significant other are considered unacceptable.

Regardless of the path that a current candidate has chosen to take to fulfill the requirements for eligibility to take the NATABOC certification examination, the following basic requirements must be met in order to apply:

* Proof of graduation from an accredited college or university.
* Proof of current CPR certification and first aid card.
* The candidate must verify that he or she has satisfied 25% of the mandatory field experience hours in practice or game coverage situations. These hours must involve one or more high-risk or high-contact sports such as football, ice hockey, gymnastics, etc.
* An approved curriculum candidate may apply to take the certification examination prior to graduation as long as he or she has completed all the required academic and clinical requirements outlined by the NATABOC. The examination may be taken on the test date that is the closest to the candidate's anticipated date of graduation.
* An internship candidate may apply to take the certification examination prior to graduation only with written verification of the intent to graduate from the dean or department chairperson of the college or university from which the candidate has been attending classes and will graduate. If the applicant has not yet completed all the mandatory academic coursework, he or she must obtain a letter of verification from the office of the registrar to prove he or she is currently enrolled in the required classes.
* Written endorsement of the candidate's application by a NATABOC athletic trainer.

To obtain an examination application, you should contact the NATABOC offices by telephone (402-559-0091) or by mail (1512 South 60th Street, Omaha, NE 68106). An application may also be obtained from the NATABOC web site at www.nataboc.org.

It is advisable to request an application 5 months prior to the examination so you have plenty of time to make sure you have all your requirements completed, any necessary forms are properly filled out, and are submitted in a timely fashion. Your test date and site will be assigned on a first-come, first-serve basis. We also suggest that you become an NATA member if you have not done so, as it will impact your application fee. The fee must be paid by check or money order and will cost **less** if you are a NATA member. Be sure to check with the NATABOC for current application fees. Be sure to send in your application at least 1 month prior to your test date to make sure it is received and accepted. If you must postpone or cancel your test for any reason, you must request this in writing at least 30 days prior to your exam date in order for you to receive a 75% refund of the examination fee. Fifty percent of the examination fee will be refunded to you if you cancel after the deadline date or you do not appear for the test. If you wish to reschedule your test date, a $100 rescheduling fee will be charged.

DEVELOPMENT OF THE NATABOC CERTIFICATION EXAMINATION

The development and administration of the NATABOC certification examination is the sole responsibility of the NATABOC, Inc. This private, nonprofit organization is governed by an eight-member board of directors consisting of five athletic trainers, a physician director, a public director, and a corporate/educational director. Within the organizational structure of the NATABOC are seven committees, each responsible for addressing various areas that are pertinent to the function of the NATABOC. Two of these committees, the Examination Administration Committee and the Examination Development Committee, are directly involved in the procedural aspects and design/validation of the examination. The questions for the test are developed, validated, and edited by certified athletic trainers. These questions are scrutinized to meet the specifications of the Role Delineation Study that was validated by the NATABOC in 1994. Once this process is completed, the approved questions are sent to Columbia Assessment Services, Inc. for additional grammatical editing and review. All the test questions developed for all three sections of the examination are based on the five domains of athletic training (prevention of athletic injuries, recognition and evaluation, rehabilitation of athletic injuries, health care administration, and professional development and responsibility).

THE NATABOC CERTIFICATION EXAMINATION FORMAT

The first certification examination given by the NATA in 1967 included 150 written questions and a practical section consisting of five questions. The original test was administered and manually scored by three athletic trainers. The certification examination has come a long way since that time and has experienced numerous changes. Currently, the test consists of three separate sections: the written section, the written simulation section, and the practical section. The examination is scored by computer, although additional precautions are taken by the testing center to ensure the test scores are accurate (eg, hand-scoring random tests and rescanning tests).

The Written Section

This section of the certification examination is a standard, 150 multiple-choice question examination based on the five domains of athletic training as identified by the Role Delineation Study validated in 1994. The questions randomly represent each domain and are worth one point each. Since there will only be one correct answer for each question, if you are unsure of an answer, we advise that you make an educated guess because your answer may be correct. You will not be penalized in this section for guessing. If you leave an answer unmarked, or you choose an incorrect answer, a point will be deducted from your score.

Five different question formats have been used:

1. The basic A-type question with five possible correct answer choices.
2. "Not" type questions, in which all the answers are correct except for one (eg, "Which of the following muscles are not located in the upper extremity?").
3. "Except" type questions, in which all the answers are correct except for one (eg, "All of the following are good sources of vitamin A except:").
4. Completion questions in which a blank word or words must be filled into the stem statement to make it correct (eg, "The two primary movements of the knee joint are _____ and _____.").
5. Multiple-correct type questions in which you must pick all of the available correct choices of those presented and equate them to the list of correct answers.

An example of a multiple-correct type question might look like this:

Which of the following are included in the classification of drugs known as NSAIDs?
I.   Motrin   IV. Indocin
II. Proventil   V. Naprosyn
III. Dilantin

A. I, II, III
B. I, III, IV, V
C. I, IV, V
D. III, IV, V

In this case, "C" would be the correct answer because Motrin, Indocin, and Naprosyn are all NSAIDs.

Many of the questions will require you to recall information (eg, a specific fact), know a definition, or apply what you know about a particular subject to a situation or condition. For example, a sample question could be:

An athlete has weak shoulder flexors. Which of the following upper extremity PNF patterns would be appropriate to strengthen this muscle group?
A. D1 flexion
B. D2 extension
C. D3 flexion
D. Contract-relax

The answer would be "A," because a D1 flexion PNF pattern incorporates shoulder flexion.

For others you will have to analyze information presented in a question and come to a conclusion based on how the parts of the question relate to each other (eg, an athlete presents with a certain problem or condition and you must assess the situation).

The questions in this manual are reflective of each area of study; they are not meant to represent the full scope of the questions that will be covered in the examination. We have presented the multiple choice section with four options/answers for reasons of economy. Please keep in mind that on the actual examination, there will be five answers offered.

This section of the examination has a 3-hour time limit, which means you cannot spend more than 1 minute per question. Work at a steady pace, but do not rush. Sometime during the written test, your name will be called and you will be escorted to the practical portion of the examination by a certified athletic trainer. Once you have completed the practical section, you will be escorted back to the testing area to finish the written examination.

When you feel satisfied that you have completed the written examination to the best of your ability, quickly scan your answer sheet to make sure you did not miss anything and check to be sure your answers correlate with the right questions. One missed answer can throw off your whole answer sheet. We also suggest you erase any unintentional marks you may have made on your answer sheet, as they may affect your score. You may leave the testing area once you are done or if the proctor announces the end of the examination period.

The Written Simulation Section

The written simulation is a unique section of the certification examination in that it requires you to become more interactive and challenges your professional judgment and problem-solving skills. This type of examination presents realistic scenarios in which you will have to make critical decisions regarding your care plan for the athlete. As you go through each scenario, you will have to make decisions regarding which actions are of immediate priority to ensure the athlete is properly cared for. As you continue through the sections of each scenario, additional information will be revealed to you, allowing you to process what is happening and make a decision on what steps you should follow next.

As mentioned earlier, you will be provided with a problem booklet, an answer booklet, and a latent-image pen for this examination. The problem booklet contains the scenario you are faced with and a selection of possible actions you have to choose from. You will decide on your answers and mark them with the latent-image pen in your answer booklet. Each answer is revealed as you make your response with the pen. A double asterisk designates the end of each answer. The answer booklet will be blank except for a list of numbers. To highlight your answers, you must highlight your response from the number toward the right until you reach the double asterisk. Do not scrub the pen against the page of the booklet, as you may mismark an answer by accident and highlight an answer you did not intend to highlight. You might also put a hole in your booklet if you rub too hard. Once an answer is marked it cannot be changed, so keep the latent pen away from your answer booklet when it is not in use. When answering questions in this part of the examination, keep in mind there is a process involved here, so only select answers that you believe are an immediate priority in solving the dilemma at hand. Follow any directions given if applicable. Make sure you carefully read through all of the possible actions first before you begin to prioritize them. This will help to minimize the chance of your making a mistake by missing an appropriate treatment option.

The written simulation is scored in a different fashion than any other part of the certification examination. Unlike the written examination, there is a penalty if you select an answer that is not appropriate for that situation or if all the correct answers are not selected. Each answer is assigned a positive point, no point (or zero), or a negative point value. There is a possible 50 points that may be scored for those answers that are correct and a possible 50 points that could be deducted from your total score for those answers that are incorrect. Neutral actions result in a zero point score and have no effect on your total score. It is not necessary to actually highlight the answers in the correct order for you to score points, but it is best if you approach your responses exactly how you would in a real-life situation, as it will increase your chances of being right. If you have specific questions concerning how the written simulation is scored, it is advised that you contact the NATABOC. You will be given 2.5 hours to finish the eight questions presented for the written simulation examination.

The Practical Section

The practical portion of the certification examination is designed to test your ability to apply your manual skills in an environment in which time and accuracy are significant factors in successfully completing the task. The room captain will ask you questions and you will be required to perform a specific task in reference to that question. You will be called during your written examination to take the practical portion and escorted to the test room by the model. This individual has been instructed not to talk about any portion of the examination as you are being escorted, so do not be offended if he or she does not answer you if you ask a question that might relate to the examination. You will bring your answer sheets with you and give them to the room captain. There will be a table in the room that will have various materials/supplies you can use during the examination. You will be instructed to examine these supplies so you know what is available for your use. You will be given a booklet that contains the questions that you will answer and be asked to read them to yourself as the examiners read the questions out loud. Your test will be tape-recorded by the room captain so you and the NATABOC will have a record of the test.

Because the examination does not begin until you begin demonstrating a task on the model or verbally acknowledge you have begun, take some time after each question is read by the examiner to plan out what you are going to do. If you do not understand a question, you may ask to have it reread to you. The model has been instructed not to talk to you or help you in any way. He or she is only there for you to demonstrate on. If the room captain feels you did not understand the question or your response is way off, he or she will stop you and repeat the question. It is wise to stop and take a second to regroup (take a deep breath!) and think of what you are doing. Think it through to make sure you have not forgotten something or made a mistake and continue to the best of your knowledge. If you finish before the allotted time is up, recheck your performance to be sure you covered everything you wanted to cover. Be sure to explain what you are doing as you demonstrate each task.

In general, you may be asked questions regarding taping/splinting or wrapping techniques, athletic training evaluation skills (such as special tests, sensory testing, checking for vital signs, goniometric measurements, or manual muscle testing, etc), rehabilitation techniques (such as PNF, mobilization techniques, etc), and treatment procedures. It is best to practice these techniques not only on other candidates, but also on certified athletic trainers who can give you constructive feedback. Use a stopwatch or clock to time yourself, since you will be under a time limit during the exam. You will be given 3 to 5 minutes to perform a taping/wrapping technique and 8 to 10 minutes for any other task.

Points are scored as you answer the question and demonstrate all the necessary steps. You will lose a point if you do not perform the task in the allotted time, but you will not be given additional credit for completing a specific task before your time is up. Make sure you demonstrate and explain your technique thoroughly, but only do what is necessary to answer the question; and when evaluating and testing on the model, be sure to perform all your evaluations in a sequence and demonstrate your special tests bilaterally.

Chapter III

Written Examination Sample Questions

Athletic Training Domains

Prevention of Athletic Injury and Illness

1. A sphygmomanometer is a device that measures which of the following?
   A. Grip strength
   B. Body fat percentage
   C. Intra-abdominal pressure
   D. None of the above

2. A Q-angle of >25° may predispose an athlete to what postural deviation?
   A. Excessive genu varus
   B. Excessive genu valgus
   C. Genu recurvatum
   D. Coxa valgus

3. What position is the "recommended" position for manually muscle testing the gluteus medius muscle?
   A. Sidelying, with the affected limb on top
   B. Supine
   C. Prone
   D. Sitting

4. All of the following are factors in lower extremity overuse syndromes in runners **except:**
   A. Poor footwear
   B. Poor posture
   C. Change in surface
   D. Short strides

5. What is the average range of motion of knee flexion?
   A. 0° to 135°
   B. 0° to 120°
   C. 0° to 100°
   D. 0° to 155°

6. All of the following questions are significant when screening a young athlete for an underlying cardiac abnormality **except**:
   A. Does the athlete have chest pain with activity?
   B. Does the athlete have a family history of sudden cardiac death in a family member under age 50?
   C. Does the athlete have numbness or tingling in either or both hands in cold weather?
   D. Does the athlete have a history of a "racing heart"?

7. True leg length discrepancy is measured between which two points?
   A. The posterior inferior iliac spine to the medial malleolus
   B. The umbilicus to the mid-patella
   C. The umbilicus to the lateral malleolus
   D. The anterior superior iliac spine to the medial malleolus

8. What position should the athlete be in to manually muscle test the hip flexors, and where should the athletic trainer's force be directed during testing?
   A. Prone, with the force directed down onto the posterior thigh
   B. Sidelying, with the force directed down onto the side of the thigh
   C. Sitting, with the force directed down onto the anterior aspect of the thigh
   D. Sitting, with the force directed down onto the medial aspect of the thigh

9. To manually muscle test the deltoids, what position should the athlete's shoulder be in?
   A. Abducted to 0° and externally rotated to 45°
   B. Abducted to 90°
   C. Flexed with the palm down
   D. Extended with the palm up

10. An abnormal lateral curvature of the vertebral column is known as what?
    A. Kyphosis
    B. Spondylolysis
    C. Scoliosis
    D. Lordosis

11. During your evaluation of an athlete's shoulder, you notice his left scapula is "winging." What is this indicative of?
    A. Rhomboid weakness
    B. Deltoid weakness
    C. Serratus anterior weakness
    D. Upper trapezius weakness

12. Bracing for scoliosis of the spine may be effective with all ages **except**:
    A. 5 year olds
    B. 10 year olds
    C. 18 year olds
    D. 14 year olds

13. During a preparticipation physical, the team physician comes across a basketball player with the following profile: The athlete is tall with an arm span greater than his height, pectus carinatum or excavatum, high-arched palate and myopia.
    What is the probable diagnosis?
    A. Paget's disease
    B. Milch disease
    C. Marfan's syndrome
    D. Gigantism

14. An athlete's pulmonary function is tested via spirometry. Several measurements are taken during this test. The maximum amount of air that can be expired after a maximum inspiration is known as:
    A. Maximum expiratory flow rate
    B. Forced expiratory volume
    C. Vital capacity
    D. Tidal volume

15. During a preparticipation exam, an athlete is diagnosed with myopia. What is this athlete's problem?
    A. Double vision
    B. Farsightedness
    C. Blindness in one eye
    D. Nearsightedness

16. All of the following are functions of the liver **except**:
    A. Carbohydrate metabolism
    B. Detoxification of blood
    C. Protein synthesis
    D. Detoxification of urine

17. The maximal rate at which oxygen is consumed and utilized while exercising is known as the maximal oxygen consumption or VO_2 max. What is the normal range of VO_2 max for an average college athlete?
    A. 80 to 100 mL/kg/min
    B. 45 to 60 mL/kg/min
    C. 70 to 80 mL/kg/min
    D. 45 to 60 dL/g/min

18. Which of the following is an indirect method of monitoring oxygen consumption?
    A. Measuring respiratory rate
    B. Measuring vital capacity
    C. Drawing blood gases during testing
    D. None of the above

19. During exercise, the body's oxygen stores are greatly diminished. The recovery O_2 is used for all the following **except**:
    A. Replace O_2 dissolved in tissue fluids
    B. Return muscle myoglobin to resting values
    C. Increase venous oxyhemoglobin to pre-exercise levels
    D. Return the catecholamine level to normal in the blood

20. All of the following functions contribute to the athlete's ability to maintain a steady state during periods of increased metabolic needs during exercise **except**:
    A. Pulmonary diffusion
    B. Vascular adaptation
    C. Physical condition of the involved muscles
    D. A high-protein pre-event meal

21. Submaximal exercise tests, which evaluate physical working capacity (PWC) by measuring heart rate increases with exercise, include all of the following **except**:
    A. Progressive pulse rate test
    B. Harvard step test
    C. Cooper 12-minute run-walk test
    D. The Saltin-Astrand VO_2 debt test

22. One method of estimating body fat has been through the use of skin-fold measurements. These four sites include all of the following **except**:
    A. Biceps
    B. Triceps
    C. Suprailiac
    D. Suprascapular

23. In hot, wet environments, the athlete's ability to adjust to a significantly increased cardiovascular workload is limited by which factor?
    A. Hypoxia
    B. Hypervolemia
    C. Dehydration
    D. Inability to dissipate heat by evaporation

24. When testing the physical conditioning of an athlete, the coach asks the athlete to sprint 50 yards. What does this test the athlete for?
    A. Aerobic endurance
    B. Vital capacity
    C. Lower extremity power
    D. Anaerobic capacity

25. What is the definition of power?
    A. Power = work x force
    B. Power = speed x distance
    C. Power = force x distance
    D. Power = work x velocity

26. During prolonged, intense training and conditioning of an athlete, what cardiac change may occur over a period of time?
    A. Development of heart murmurs
    B. Development of PVCs
    C. Increase in heart size
    D. Decrease in heart size

27. If it was determined that a 25-year-old athlete should work at 80% of his maximal heart rate, at what would the target heart rate be calculated?
    A. 170 BPM
    B. 156 BPM
    C. 145 BPM
    D. 140 BPM

28. What period of time does it take during a "warm-up" to adequately prepare the body for athletic performance?
    A. 5 to 10 minutes
    B. 35 to 45 minutes
    C. 60 minutes
    D. 15 to 30 minutes

29. On the average, an athlete expends between _____ to _____ calories per day.
    A. 4000 to 5000
    B. 2000 to 3000
    C. 2500 to 3000
    D. 2200 to 4400

30. An athlete's diet should consist of approximately _____ protein, _____ fat, and _____ carbohydrate.
    A. 12% to 15%, 40% to 50%, 55% to 70%
    B. 10% to 20%, 30% to 40%, 50% to 70%
    C. 5% to 10%, 30% to 45%, 60% to 80%
    D. 25% to 35%, 55% to 65%, 70% to 90%

31. The pre-event meal should be planned by whom?
    A. The coach
    B. The athlete
    C. The athletic trainer
    D. The athlete, athletic trainer, and coach

32. What is the minimum amount of time needed prior to an event to digest a meal?
    A. 2 to 3 hours
    B. 3 to 4 hours
    C. 5 to 6 hours
    D. 6 to 8 hours

33. How many glasses of water should an athlete consume on a daily basis?
    A. No more than 8
    B. 2 to 3
    C. 8 or more
    D. 5 to 7

34. In female athletes with inconsistent menstrual cycles, adequate calcium intake is essential. How much calcium should the athlete consume a day?
    A. 500 to 700 mg
    B. 750 mg
    C. 1000 mg
    D. 1500 mg

35. When monitoring a carbohydrate-loading program for an endurance athlete, what should the athlete do the day prior to competition?
    A. Eat a high-carbohydrate meal and perform little or no exercise
    B. Eat a low-carbohydrate meal and participate in a regular amount of exercise
    C. Eat a high-carbohydrate meal and participate in a regular amount of exercise
    D. Hyperhydrate and rest the day before competition

36. The major side effect of the NSAID group is:
    A. Vertigo
    B. Tinnitus
    C. Drowsiness
    D. Gastrointestinal upset

37. Your athlete is on a medication for a staph aureus infection. Which of the following adverse reactions might you expect with antibiotic treatment?
    A. Palpitations
    B. Abdominal cramping
    C. Dry mouth
    D. Headache

38. The normal dosage for one tablet of aspirin is:
    A. 325 mg
    B. 400 mg
    C. 500 mg
    D. 375 mg

39. All of the following are possible side effects of oral contraceptives **except**:
    A. Nausea and vomiting
    B. Shortness of breath
    C. Fluid retention
    D. Amenorrhea

40. Anabolic steroids are often abused by athletics. Which of the following results may occur in the female athlete after ingesting testosterone?
    A. Decreased libido
    B. Gynecomastia
    C. Hirsutism
    D. Increased body fat

41. Ultrasound is based on the _____ effect.
    A. Resonance
    B. Sounding
    C. Reverse piezoelectric
    D. Phoresor

42. What medium does **not** transmit ultrasound waves?
    A. Water
    B. Air
    C. Body lotion
    D. Steroid creams

43. What kind of heating method does a warm whirlpool utilize?
    A. Conduction
    B. Convection
    C. Radiation
    D. Evaporation

44. The term used in ultrasound to describe the time that sound waves are being emitted during one pulse period is:
    A. Ultrasound frequency
    B. Cavitation
    C. Attenuation
    D. Duty cycle

45. A moist heat pack is what kind of heater?
    A. Superficial
    B. Deep
    C. Cutaneous
    D. Surface

46. "Conventional TENS" uses a frequency in the _____ PPS range with a phase duration of _____ μseconds.
    A. 50 to 100, 250
    B. 50 to 100, 2 to 50
    C. 2 to 4, >150
    D. >100, 20 to 30

47. One of the most serious adverse reactions during iontophoresis treatment is:
    A. Galvanic burns
    B. Anaphylactic shock
    C. Dermatitis
    D. Histamine reaction

48. Paraffin bath therapy is commonly used on the hands and feet as a method of superficial heating. To keep the paraffin mixture in a molten state, the temperature should be maintained between:
    A. 100° to 115° F
    B. 80° to 105° F
    C. 126° to 130° F
    D. 118° to 125° F

49. The therapeutic conversion of electrical energy into high-frequency sound energy above the audible range to create heat in the tissues is the definition of what modality?
    A. Diathermy
    B. Ultrasound
    C. Electric stimulation
    D. TENS

50. Ultrasound waves are reflected by _____ and absorbed by _____.
    A. Bone, skin
    B. Skin, connective tissue
    C. Skin, blood
    D. Bone, muscle

51. Which of the below are contraindications to massage?
    I.   Inflammation   IV. Infection
    II. Pregnancy   V. Phlebitis
    III. Hemorrhage

    A. I, II, III, IV
    B. I, III, IV, V
    C. II, III, IV
    D. II, III, IV, V

52. Which of the following is not an indication for diathermy?
    A. To increase local circulation
    B. Reduction of spasms
    C. Pain relief
    D. Cardiac abnormalities

53. Which of the following is not a contraindication or precaution for the use of ultrasound?
    A. Scarring
    B. Acute hemorrhage
    C. Anesthesia
    D. Treating over the endocrine gland

54. Which physical law is applied with the use of an infrared lamp?
    A. Joule's law
    B. Inverse square law
    C. Wolff's law
    D. Ohm's law

55. _____ and _____ are two means by which to deliver medication via sound waves and electricity.
    A. Ultrasound, iontophoresis
    B. Ultrasound, phonophoresis
    C. Micromassage, phonophoresis
    D. Phonophoresis, iontophoresis

56. What is a primary indication for cervical traction?
    A. Muscle spasm
    B. Hemorrhage
    C. Muscle weakness
    D. Vertigo

57. When working on a bleeding athlete, the athletic trainer should always:
    A. Avoid touching the bloody areas
    B. Wash hands before treatment
    C. Wear latex gloves
    D. Wear eye protection

58. Alpine skiing world championships are scheduled in Japan. Jet lag is bound to occur as a result of crossing several time zones. What should the athletic trainer recommend to the team members prior to their flight to combat the jet lag effect?
    A. Upon arrival, adjust all training, eating, and sleeping schedules to the local time of the country in which they are competing
    B. Consume caffeine only when traveling east
    C. Reset watches to the new time zone 3 days in advance to get used to the time change
    D. When traveling west, it is important to have a large breakfast in the morning to carry the athlete through the day

59. During a football practice in early September, the temperature is measured and found to be between 90° to 100° F, but the humidity is under 70%. What should the athletic trainer recommend to the football staff?
    A. Suspend practice for the day
    B. Keep a careful watch on any athlete who is grossly overweight
    C. Have the athletes take a 10-minute rest every hour and change t-shirts when wet
    D. Limit practice to 30 minutes

60. What is the best way to prevent otitis externa?
    A. Avoid contact activities for 7 to 10 days
    B. Use ear plugs during activity
    C. Dry the external auditory canal after swimming
    D. Wear adequate protective devices for the ear

61. How is pediculosis spread between individuals?
    A. Coughing and sneezing
    B. Poor hand washing/hygiene
    C. Close sexual contact
    D. Contact with open sores

62. When fitting the athlete with protective equipment, what factors should be considered?
    A. Athlete's skill level
    B. Athlete's size
    C. Sport position
    D. All of the above

63. Which of the steps below are correct when fitting a football helmet?
    I.   Place the helmet over the head, tilt it backward, rotate it forward into position
    II. Try to turn helmet side to side with the head in a stationary position
    III. Check to make sure the helmet sits three finger-breadths above the eyebrows
    IV. Press straight down on the crown of the helmet to see if the pressure is at the crown of the head
    V.   Check to see if the jaw pads fit snugly against the jaw
    VI. Check the chin strap adjustment for a tight fit

    A. I, II, IV, V, VI
    B. I, II, III, VI
    C. I, III, IV, V
    D. I, III, IV, VI

64. All of the following conditions would disqualify an athlete from athletic competition **except**:
    A. Renal disease
    B. Uncontrolled hypertension
    C. Acute mononucleosis
    D. The absence of one testicle

65. A student athletic trainer in an internship program must be supervised by whom to perform athletic training tasks?
    A. Physician
    B. School coach
    C. Certified athletic trainer
    D. School nurse

66. Which piece of information is not part of the athletic trainer's daily documentation?
    A. Treatment technique
    B. Playing status
    C. Daily injury log
    D. Athlete's insurance information

67. All of the following are important steps in avoiding legal problems when administering care to the athlete **except**:
    A. Keeping accurate records
    B. Staying familiar with the health history of the athlete
    C. Following orders of the team physician
    D. Allowing the coach to decide when the athlete should return to play after injury

68. "Torts" are legal wrongs committed against a person or his or her property. Such wrongs may be a direct result of _____ or _____.
    A. Negligence, commission
    B. Negligence, liability
    C. Omission, commission
    D. Omission, negligence

69. The _____ and _____ should be involved with the athletic trainer in selecting and maintaining the athlete's protective equipment.
    A. Coach, team physician
    B. Coach, equipment manager
    C. Equipment manager, athlete
    D. Team physician, coach

70. Which of the following organizations certifies football helmets to make sure they are able to withstand repeated blows of high mass and low velocity?
    A. FDA
    B. NOCSAE
    C. NATA
    D. NFL

71. Football helmets may fall into one or two categories. These two types are known as _____ or _____.
    A. Air/fluid-filled, padded
    B. Gel-filled, padded
    C. Plastic, fiberglass
    D. Standard, adjustable

72. When is maximum protection provided by a properly fitting mouthguard?
    A. When it is made of a flexible, resilient material and is form-fitted to the teeth and upper jaw
    B. When it is made of a rigid, plastic material that is fitted to both the upper and lower jaw
    C. When it is NOCSAE certified
    D. When it is NCAA certified

73. Properly fitting shoulder pads should adequately cover the shoulder complex. Which structure should the epaulets and cups completely cover?
    A. The scapula
    B. The deltoids
    C. The pectoralis major
    D. The trapezius

74. A flak jacket is a piece of equipment designed to protect the athlete after what type of injury?
    A. Scapular injury
    B. Hip pointer
    C. Abdominal injury
    D. Rib injury

75. Which of the following organizations set the standards for eye protection for racquet sports?
    A. American College of Sports Medicine (ACSM)
    B. NATA
    C. FDA
    D. American Society for Testing and Materials (ASTM)

76. Of the following pieces of equipment, which is not an NCAA-mandated piece of equipment?
    A. Wrestling—ear guards
    B. Men's lacrosse—protective gloves
    C. Baseball—double ear flap helmet for batting
    D. Gymnastics—palm protectors for the uneven parallel bars

77. Which of the following is not a duty of the athletic trainer?
    A. Counsel and advise the athlete about health care
    B. Diagnose and treat injuries
    C. Administer first aid as necessary
    D. Supervise proper equipment fitting

Recognition, Evaluation, and Immediate Care of Injuries

1. A positive Thompson sign is indicative of what problem?
   A. Tight hip flexor
   B. Tight iliotibial band
   C. Ruptured Achilles' tendon
   D. Ruptured posterior tibialis tendon

2. A simple movement to check the integrity of the radial nerve would be:
   A. Elbow flexion
   B. Wrist extension
   C. Forearm supination
   D. Thumb to little finger opposition

3. A grade I ankle sprain involves which structure?
   A. Tibiofibular ligament
   B. Posterior talofibular ligament
   C. Calcaneofibular ligament
   D. Anterior talofibular ligament

4. You are covering a football game when two players collide. You notice one player grab his neck and shake his arm. When you examine him, he complains of lateral neck discomfort and a feeling of "numbness" or "burning" down his arm. His arm is hanging limp by his side. In a few minutes, the symptoms subside. What do you suspect?
   A. Carpal tunnel syndrome
   B. Long thoracic nerve injury
   C. A "burner" or pinched nerve syndrome
   D. Dorsal scapular nerve injury

5. Which test, if positive, is suspect of a torn posterior cruciate ligament?
   A. Sag sign
   B. Anterior drawer sign
   C. McMurray's sign
   D. Ober sign

6. At what point should the athletic trainer's initial evaluation of an injury begin?
   A. At the moment the injury is witnessed
   B. Once the athlete has been stabilized in the training room
   C. Once the athletic trainer receives a medical referral from a doctor
   D. After the athlete is seen by the team doctor

7. Which scale is important in assessing the severity of a head injury?
   A. Beck's Orientation Scale
   B. Glasgow Coma Scale
   C. Rancho Los Amigos Amnesia Scale
   D. Intracranial Pressure Scale

8. What quick test can be performed to check if nerve root L5 is intact?
   A. Have the athlete flex his or her hip in standing
   B. Have the athlete walk on his or her toes
   C. Have the athlete extend his or her great toe
   D. Have the athlete extend his or her hip

9. A positive Phalen's sign is suspect of what problem?
   A. Tarsal tunnel syndrome
   B. Carpal tunnel syndrome
   C. Thoracic outlet syndrome
   D. Suprascapular entrapment syndrome

10. The Trendelenburg test is a method used to evaluate the competence of what structures?
    A. Hip flexors
    B. Peroneal muscles
    C. Hip abductors
    D. Erector spinae

11. What evaluative test is used to examine the integrity of the lateral collateral ligament of the knee?
    A. Pivot shift test
    B. Valgus stress test
    C. Lachman's test
    D. Varus stress test

12. A positive drop-arm sign is indicative of:
    A. Posterior shoulder subluxation
    B. Torn rotator cuff muscle
    C. Axillary nerve injury
    D. A labral tear

13. If there is inflammation at the site of the medial epicondyle of the elbow, which of the following tests would be positive?
    A. Tennis elbow test
    B. Golfer's elbow test
    C. Tinel's test
    D. Finkelstein's test

14. All of the following are signs of an injury **except**:
    A. Change in skin color or texture
    B. Change in body temperature
    C. Change in blood pressure
    D. Complaint of headaches

15. Information gained during the palpation phase of the athletic trainer's initial assessment might include all of the following **except**:
    A. Presence of crepitus
    B. Sensory function
    C. Presence of a deformity
    D. Degree of functional movement

16. During an upper quarter screen, checking the strength of thumb extension correlates to what nerve root?
    A. T1
    B. C8
    C. C5
    D. C4

17. A positive "clunk" test is indicative of what pathology?
    A. Unstable ankle
    B. Olecranon fracture
    C. Meniscus tear of the knee
    D. Glenoid labrum tear

18. A baseball player comes to see the athletic trainer and is complaining of diffuse pain, clicking, and a sensation of "slipping" of his right shoulder when throwing. What pathology might the athletic trainer suspect with this type of presentation?
    A. Torn rotator cuff
    B. Thrower's exostosis
    C. A-C joint pathology
    D. Labral pathology

19. Two major symptoms of a spontaneous pneumothorax include _____ and _____.
    A. Bradycardia, cyanosis
    B. Sudden chest pain, dyspnea
    C. Apnea with rales, rhonchi
    D. Left shoulder pain, cyanosis

20. The _____ pulse and _____ pulse should be palpated after an acute traumatic injury to the knee area to make sure the peripheral circulation to the involved limb is adequate.
    A. Posterior tibial, dorsalis pedis
    B. Anterior tibial, plantar
    C. Saphenous, dorsalis pedis
    D. Femoral, posterior tibial

21. Foot drop may be indicative of what pathology?
    A. Plantar nerve injury
    B. Shin splints
    C. Peroneal nerve injury
    D. Achilles' tendinitis

22. A type V Salter fracture involves what kind of fracture through the physeal plate?
    A. The epiphysis and metaphysis separate without fragmentation
    B. A crush injury to the epiphysis
    C. The epiphysis and metaphysis separate with fragmentation
    D. The epiphysis, metaphysis, and physis all separate from each other

23. An athlete you have just evaluated for a possible head injury has a noticeable facial droop on the left side of his face. Which cranial nerve(s) is involved?
    A. I
    B. IV, V
    C. VII
    D. III, IX

24. During your examination of an athlete who has been complaining of weakness when using the rowing machine in the weight room, you notice his right latissimus dorsi muscle appears atrophied. Which nerve is affected?
    A. Trigeminal nerve
    B. Thoracodorsal nerve
    C. Dorsoscapular nerve
    D. Thoracic spinal nerve

25. A second-degree burn will have which of the following characteristics?
    A. A raised, reddened appearance
    B. A white, mottled appearance
    C. A blackened, hard appearance
    D. A reddened area with blisters

26. The athlete may have difficulty performing what actions if the medial and lateral pectoral nerves are injured?
    A. Flexion, adduction, and internal rotation of the upper arm
    B. Shoulder shrugs
    C. Abduction and external rotation of the upper arm
    D. Extension, internal rotation, and adduction of the upper arm

27. A gymnast reports to the athletic trainer with a complaint of low back pain, which has been present for approximately 1 week. After being sent to the doctor for evaluation, a "Scotty dog" defect is seen on x-ray. This finding confirms which condition?
    A. Fractured transverse process of a vertebrae
    B. Fractured demifacet of a vertebrae
    C. Spondylolisthesis
    D. Spondylolysis

28. An athlete is poked in the eye with a finger and comes to the athletic trainer for evaluation. He is having significant difficulty opening his eye. Which of the following muscles might have sustained an injury?
     A. Levator capitis inferioris
     B. Splenius capitus
     C. Levator palpebrae superioris
     D. Levator palpebrae orbitis

29. An athlete is brought to the training room after being struck in the back of the head with a bat by accident. He is complaining of blurred vision. Which part of the brain has been affected?
     A. Frontal lobe
     B. Parietal lobe
     C. Temporal lobe
     D. Occipital lobe

30. What internal organ is diseased if the athlete presents with jaundice?
     A. Spleen
     B. Pancreas
     C. Gallbladder
     D. Liver

31. Which two structures are injured with a Bankart lesion?
     A. Anterior capsule of the shoulder and the glenoid labrum
     B. The inferior capsule of the shoulder and glenoid fossa
     C. The articular surface of the humeral head and glenoid labrum
     D. The surgical neck of the humerus and the coracoacromial ligament

32. An athlete has a wrist injury that is limiting his ability to supinate his forearm. In what plane of motion does supination and pronation of the forearm take place?
     A. Frontal
     B. Horizontal
     C. Sagittal
     D. Vertical

33. The sensation that an athlete might experience just prior to an epileptic seizure is called:
     A. An aura
     B. A hallucination
     C. A delusion
     D. Pre-epileptic vertigo

34. The inflammatory process includes all of the following signs and symptoms **except**:
     A. Redness
     B. Pain
     C. Warmth
     D. Numbness

35. Changes in blood pressure may occur as a result of many factors. Two of these factors may include _____ and _____.
    A. Exercise, change in posture
    B. Change in posture, respiratory rate
    C. Level of consciousness, body size
    D. Respiratory rate, pH levels of the blood

36. Type I diabetes is characterized by an impaired capacity to secrete insulin due to a beta cell defect. This type of diabetes is commonly seen in what type of individual?
    A. Obese, geriatric
    B. Lean, insulin dependent
    C. Noninsulin dependent, obese
    D. Noninsulin dependent, juvenile

37. All of the following are true about infectious mononucleosis **except**:
    A. The attack rate is highest between 15- to 25-years-olds
    B. The virus is excreted in saliva
    C. The primary symptom is low back pain
    D. It is caused by transmission of the Epstein-Barr virus

38. Which of the following is the organism that is one of the most common causes of vaginitis in women?
    A. AIDS
    B. Genital herpes
    C. Chlamydia trachomatis
    D. Candida

39. All of the following are risk factors for osteoporosis **except**:
    A. Early menopause
    B. High consumption of alcohol, cigarettes, and caffeine
    C. Sedentary lifestyle
    D. Obesity

40. An athlete with an infection or serious disease such as leukemia might demonstrate an abnormally raised white blood cell count. What is the normal leukocyte count?
    A. 200,000 to 400,000/cu mm
    B. 500 to 1500/cu mm
    C. 4000 to 10,000/cu mm
    D. 1000 to 40,000/cu mm

41. What is the primary target of the AIDS virus in the body?
    A. Neutrophils
    B. Basophils
    C. T-helper lymphocytes
    D. Phagocytes

42. EIA stands for what clinical entity?
    A. Exercise-induced arrhythmia
    B. Exercise-induced asthma
    C. Exercise-induced allergy
    D. Exercise-induced aneurysm

43. What type of gait deviation might the athletic trainer see with an athlete who has sustained an ankle injury and has decreased range of motion in dorsiflexion?
    A. Lateral trunk bending
    B. Trendelenburg gait
    C. Hip hiking
    D. Wide walking base

44. A soccer player has fractured his right lower leg and has been placed in a cast and given crutches. The addition of crutches does what to his center of gravity?
    A. Moves it to the left
    B. Moves it to the mid-abdominal area
    C. Moves it to the right
    D. Just enlarges the base of support

45. You notice one of your gymnasts has lost a significant amount of weight over the last month. She is always concerned about her image when she discusses her performance with you. What might you suspect as the problem?
    A. Drug dependence
    B. Depression
    C. Narcissism
    D. Anorexia nervosa

46. An athlete who sustains a severe or career-ending injury may go through a progression of emotional reactions, which are frequently seen with an individual who has experienced a significant loss. All of the following are included in this series of reactions **except**:
    A. Guilt
    B. Anger
    C. Acceptance
    D. Denial

47. All of the following are symptoms of an overtrained athlete **except**:
    A. Emotional lability
    B. Loss of appetite
    C. Reduced concentration
    D. Excessive motivation

48. Which of the following signs/symptoms are present in a depressed athlete?
    A. Decreased appetite
    B. Insomnia
    C. Fatigue
    D. All of the above

49. The athletic trainer notices one of the baseball players routinely cleans his cleats after every game and practice so no dirt is visible, and he checks his equipment bag multiple times to assure himself his "lucky towel" is with him. This is an example of what type of behavior?
    A. Schizophrenic
    B. Anxiety
    C. Obsessive-compulsive
    D. Passive-aggressive

50. All of the following are possible factors regarding why an athlete might be injury prone **except**:
    A. Bad luck
    B. Problems at home
    C. Joint hypermobility
    D. Poor endurance

51. Results of severe fluid restriction during weight loss attempts by a wrestler may include:
    A. Higher resting heart rate
    B. Increased renal flow
    C. Increased stroke volume
    D. Higher O_2 consumption

52. What is wrong with the athlete eating a 12- to 16-ounce steak, baked potato, scrambled eggs, and coffee with sugar 4 hours prior to an event?
    A. Coffee with sugar may take as long as 3 hours to metabolize
    B. The intestinal tract will be full at the time of competition because it is a large meal
    C. The athlete may be hungry 8 hours later after he or she competes
    D. Nothing; the pre-event meal should be at least 500 calories or more

53. What happens when an athlete consumes a simple sugar prior to an event?
    A. May cause a sudden decrease in blood glucose because of a sudden increase in insulin production
    B. May lead to a sudden increase in blood glucose because of a decrease in insulin production
    C. May lead to increased blood levels of electrolytes
    D. May lead to hyperlipidemia

54. Which is not a good source of vitamin C?
    A. Broccoli
    B. Strawberries
    C. Oranges
    D. Nuts

55. A female gymnast is complaining of symptoms of PMS (premenstrual syndrome) such as irritability, anxiety, depression, and bloating. Which of the following vitamins might be helpful in alleviating these symptoms?
    A. Vitamin B6
    B. Vitamin B12
    C. Vitamin K
    D. Vitamin A

56. While discussing general nutrition principles with a female swimmer who is a strict vegetarian, the athletic trainer should be aware that her diet might lack what mineral?
    A. Choline
    B. Iron
    C. Niacin
    D. Folate

57. Which type of drink would **not** be appropriate prior to a long-distance run?
    A. Water
    B. Regular cola soda
    C. Gatorade
    D. Water with lemon juice added

58. A megadose of which of the following vitamins is potentially very dangerous?
    A. Vitamin A
    B. Vitamin B1
    C. Vitamin C
    D. Vitamin B2

59. An athlete informs the athletic trainer that he is taking tetracycline for a respiratory infection. Tetracycline will bind with which of the following two minerals to form a nonabsorbable complex (and therefore should **not** be taken before meals)?
    A. Potassium and zinc
    B. Sodium and magnesium
    C. Iron and calcium
    D. Iron and phosphorus

60. In general, what percent body fat is a healthy range for a female athlete?
    A. 20% to 25%
    B. 15% to 30%
    C. 5% to 10%
    D. 12% to 14%

61. A loss of water equaling what percent of body weight will begin to threaten athletic performances?
    A. 2% to 3%
    B. 0.5% to 1%
    C. 1% to 2%
    D. 1% to 1.5%

62. Which of the following medications is **not** an NSAID?
    A. Aspirin
    B. Motrin
    C. Tylenol
    D. Orudis KT

63. All of the following drugs may be used with phonophoresis during the acute phase of treatment **except:**
    A. Dexamethasone
    B. Hydrocortisone
    C. Lidocaine
    D. Naproxen

64. Which of the following medications is **not** an antihistamine drug?
    A. Dimetapp
    B. Ultram
    C. Benadryl
    D. Claritin

65. An athlete comes to your office complaining of intense itching and burning pain between his toes and he cannot find anything to help alleviate the symptoms. The area is reddened with some white flakes. What might you recommend?
    A. Neosporin ointment
    B. Tinactin spray
    C. Silvadene cream
    D. Eucerin cream

66. One of your athletes has been diagnosed with psoriasis. All of the following medications are appropriate for treatment of this condition **except**:
    A. Aristocort
    B. Kenalog
    C. Topicort
    D. Betadine

67. Which of the following is **not** a medication that is delivered via a metered-dose inhaler for EIA?
    A. Proventil
    B. Alupent
    C. Butisol
    D. Ventolin

68. What medication is often used for anxiety or panic attacks?
    A. Zantac
    B. Xanax
    C. Thorazine
    D. Prozac

69. What is the primary mode of action of penicillin?
    A. Increases the number of T-lymphocytes in the bloodstream
    B. Inhibits the metabolism of the bacteria
    C. Prevents bacterial reproduction
    D. Breaks down the cell wall of the bacteria

70. If the athlete complains of a burning sensation during an ultrasound treatment, all of the following may be the source of the problem **except**:
    A. The intensity is too high
    B. Not enough ultrasound medium is being used
    C. Too much ultrasound gel is being used
    D. The movement of the transducer head is too slow

71. Which of the following is considered a medical emergency?
    A. Acute compartment syndrome
    B. Navicular fracture
    C. Bulimia
    D. Mitral valve prolapse

72. All of the following treatments would be inappropriate for an acute quadriceps contusion **except**:
    A. Light massage
    B. Pulsed ultrasound
    C. Ice massage followed by gentle stretch
    D. Ice pack with compression wrap with the knee in flexion

73. Deep frostbite is a medical emergency. What would the proper course of treatment be for this problem?
    A. Very slow, careful rewarming of the body part with warm water
    B. Firm, sustained pressure of the hand on the affected body part
    C. Rapid rewarming of the affected body part with warm water
    D. Quick friction in order to increase local circulation

74. An athlete collides with a teammate during an ice hockey game and sustains a blow to the jaw with a hockey stick. He is holding his lower face with his hands and is in intense pain. All of the following procedures will assist the trainer in determining if there is a fracture of the jaw **except**:
    A. Have the athlete bite and observe for a malocclusion
    B. See if the athlete can retract his jaw and observe for difficulty with movement
    C. Ask the athlete to open and close his mouth, noting asymmetry with movement
    D. Palpate for jaw deformity when it is at rest, open, and closed

75. During which of the circumstances below should an athlete be immediately referred to a dentist?
    I.   The tooth is knocked out
    II. When a tooth is displaced 2 mm or more
    III. When a crown is fractured and the tooth is still alive
    IV. When a filling is knocked out or fractured and the athlete is sensitive to hot or cold food
    V.   When an artificial plate is broken during competition

    A. I, II, III
    B. I, II, III, V
    C. I, V
    D. II, III, IV

76. An athlete sustains a blunt trauma injury to the upper right quadrant of the abdomen. What structure might be injured in this area?
    A. Liver
    B. Gall bladder
    C. Spleen
    D. Pancreas

77. A male athlete sustains a direct blow to the genital area. How can the athletic trainer immediately decrease the pain?
    A. Use an ice pack to the area
    B. Use direct pressure on the testes
    C. Have the athlete lie supine with his knees bent to his chest to decrease the strain on the scrotum
    D. Have the athlete long-sit, lift him approximately 6 inches off the ground with support under the axilla and drop the athlete to the ground

78. When performing two-person CPR, what is the correct compression to breath ratio?
    A. 5:2
    B. 15:2
    C. 15:1
    D. 5:1

79. Shock after a severe injury can result from _____ or _____.
    A. Pain, increased blood pressure
    B. Decreased heart rate, infection
    C. Hemorrhage, hypothermia
    D. Hemorrhage, stagnation of blood

80. Which of the following symptoms below represent a second-degree concussion?
    I.   Blurring or loss of consciousness lasting from 20 seconds to 5 minutes
    II. Headache and amnesia are often present
    III. Athlete is often confused and disoriented
    IV. There are no positive signs on neurologic testing and examination
    V.   There is no complaint of a headache
    VI. Altered level of consciousness lasts less than 10 to 20 seconds

    A. II, IV, VI
    B. I, IV, V
    C. I, II, III
    D. IV, V, VI

81. "Cauliflower ear" is an injury to which structure of the ear?
    A. Tympanic membrane
    B. External auditory canal
    C. Pinna
    D. Eustachian tube

82. An athlete who had been diagnosed with infectious mononucleosis has just been cleared by the team doctor to return to full activity. How long should the athlete remain out of contact participation from the time of onset to the time of full recovery?
    A. 2 weeks
    B. At least 3 weeks
    C. 6 months
    D. A maximum of 6 weeks

83. What may proteinuria indicate?
    A. Pancreatitis
    B. Possible gall stones
    C. Renal or urinary tract pathology
    D. Diabetes

84. What would be the most appropriate type of roentgenogram for a possible tibial stress fracture?
    A. X-ray
    B. Bone scan
    C. MRI
    D. CT scan

85. A rugby player sustains a confirmed head injury during a game and had been removed from the game. All of the following are symptoms/signs of increasing intracerebral pressure that the athletic trainer should monitor **except**:
    A. Nausea and vomiting
    B. Pupil irregularity
    C. Increase in systolic blood pressure with decrease in diastolic blood pressure
    D. Romberg's sign

86. If an athlete is unconscious from a blow to the head, he or she should be assumed to have a neck injury in addition to a possible head injury. If the airway appears to be impaired, all of the following would be appropriate steps in management **except**:
    A. Cut the face mask with an appropriate tool and move it out of the way
    B. Leave the helmet on
    C. Stabilize the head and neck
    D. Do a finger sweep of the mouth to remove any debris and clear the airway

87. Which of the following is one of the most common eye injuries sustained in athletics?
    A. Detached iris
    B. Detached retina
    C. Zygomatic fracture
    D. Corneal abrasion

88. During the Heimlich maneuver, the athletic trainer should grasp one fist with the other hand and place the thumb side of the fist:
    A. On the abdomen between the xyphoid process and the umbilicus
    B. On the manubrium
    C. On the abdomen between the umbilicus and symphysis pubis
    D. Between the scapula

89. An athlete is brought into the training room with a 2.5 inch nail embedded in his foot. All of the following actions are appropriate in the treatment of this injury **except**:
    A. Immediately remove the nail from the foot
    B. Keep the athlete calm
    C. Pack the nail and foot as they are in a large dressing to help control the bleeding and stabilize the object
    D. Transport the athlete to the hospital with the nail still embedded in the foot

90. All of the following parameters should be assessed when checking the neurovascular status of an injured limb **except**:
    A. Sensation
    B. The pulse distal to the injury
    C. Motor function
    D. Joint range of motion

91. Which of the measures below are appropriate steps in the management of an athlete who is experiencing a seizure?
    I. Keep spectators out of the way
    II. Protect the patient's head and body from injury
    III. Turn patient on his or her side
    IV. If athlete is in status epilepticus or it is a first seizure, immediately seek additional medical support
    V. Try to keep the athlete's mouth open by any means to prevent airway obstruction
    VI. Call the athlete's next of kin to inform him or her of the problem and of the care given

    A. II, IV, V, VI
    B. I, II, III, IV
    C. II, III, IV, VI
    D. I, II, IV, V

92. A baseball player has been stung by a bee. This player has a history of a severe allergy to bee stings. A couple of minutes after being stung, the area becomes red and raised and it begins to itch. The athlete begins to complain that his tongue feels thick and he starts to have difficulty breathing. What type of shock is he beginning to develop?
    A. Neurogenic shock
    B. Metabolic shock
    C. Anaphylactic shock
    D. Respiratory shock

93. It is critical that CPR be administered as soon as possible during a life-threatening situation. If the brain is deprived of oxygen, in what amount of time is brain damage likely to occur?
    A. 0 to 4 minutes
    B. 10 to 12 minutes
    C. 4 to 6 minutes
    D. After 15 minutes

94. During CPR, it is most convenient and efficient to monitor the athlete's circulation by palpating the carotid artery. Where is the pulse located?
    A. In the groove between the larynx and the sternocleidomastoid muscle
    B. Between the mastoid process and pharynx
    C. At the base of the neck superior to the manubrium
    D. 2 inches below the base of the earlobe on the side of the neck

95. During CPR, the adult sternum must be compressed to what depth for compression to be effective?
    A. 0.5 to 1 inch
    B. 1 to 1.5 inches
    C. 1.5 to 2 inches
    D. 2 to 2.5 inches

96. Which type of heat injury is considered a medical emergency?
    A. Dehydration
    B. Heat cramps
    C. Heat stroke
    D. Heat exhaustion

97. Which of the signs and symptoms below are classical of a tension pneumothorax?
    I.   Tracheal deviation   IV. Dizziness
    II. Distended neck veins   V. Cyanosis
    III. Unilateral absence of breath sounds

    A. II, III, IV
    B. I, IV, V
    C. I, III, IV, V
    D. I, II, III, V

98. An athlete has been kicked in the low back area during a soccer game. He is complaining of significant flank pain, is having difficulty voiding, and there is blood in his urine. What should the athletic trainer suspect is injured?
    A. The kidney
    B. The large intestine
    C. The lumbar fascia
    D. The testicles

99. When evaluating an unconscious athlete, the first step the athletic trainer should take is to:
    A. Check for sources of bleeding
    B. Take vital signs
    C. Check for normal extremity movement
    D. Check to make sure the athlete's airway is open and he or she is breathing normally

100. What is the most common and devastating mechanism of injury seen in neck injuries sustained during football?
    A. Cervical hyperextension
    B. Forceful cervical lateral flexion
    C. Cervical hyperflexion and rotation
    D. Cervical hyperflexion and axial compression

101. Where would the athlete complain of pain with acute appendicitis?
    A. Lower right quadrant of the abdomen
    B. Right lateral hip area
    C. Inner right thigh
    D. Anterior right thigh area

102. What is the prudent method of transporting an athlete with a suspected spinal injury?
    A. Do not move the athlete until a doctor is present
    B. Use of a stretcher
    C. Fireman's carry
    D. Use a spine board with medical assistance

103. When fitting crutches for an athlete, the elbow should be bent to approximately:
    A. 90°
    B. 10°
    C. 30°
    D. 0°

104. After an acute musculoskeletal injury, such as a shoulder dislocation, the body releases a natural opiate-like substance, which provides temporary pain relief. What is this substance called?
     A. Prostaglandins
     B. Substance P
     C. Endorphins
     D. Insulin

105. Under what condition can CPR be stopped?
     A. If a rib is fractured during the effort
     B. The athlete vomits
     C. The athlete aspirates
     D. Not until the athletic trainer is exhausted, spontaneous respirations and pulse have returned, or a physician or another party continues CPR in place of the athletic trainer

106. After an athlete has suffered a ruptured spleen, he or she may experience pain that radiates down the left shoulder and approximately one third of the way down the upper left arm. What is this pain known as?
     A. Visceral pain
     B. Radicular pain
     C. Kehr's sign
     D. Angina

107. What would the appropriate treatment be for an athlete who has sustained a rib fracture?
     A. Use of a rib belt
     B. There is no specific treatment
     C. Total bedrest
     D. Use of a pillow to splint the ribs when coughing

108. What is the typical mechanism of injury for an anterior shoulder dislocation?
     A. Shoulder abduction with internal rotation
     B. Maximal shoulder extension
     C. Shoulder abduction with external rotation
     D. Shoulder adduction with internal rotation

109. All of the following are basic functions of athletic taping and bandaging **except**:
     A. Support of an injured body part
     B. To protect wounds from infection
     C. To enhance the athlete's skill
     D. To hold protective equipment in place

110. Taping continuously around a limb may cause what problem?
     A. Ineffective support
     B. Difficulty in tape removal
     C. Compromised circulation
     D. There is no problem with this method

111. What is the compression to breath ratio during one-person CPR?
     A. 5:1
     B. 15:2
     C. 15:1
     D. 5:2

112. Which of the symptoms below are seen with acute mountain sickness?
     I.   Insomnia   IV. Headache
     II. Vomiting   V.   Fatigue
     III. Shortness of breath with exertion

     A. II, III, IV
     B. I, III, IV, V
     C. I, II, IV, V
     D. I, II, III, V

113. An athlete reports to the athletic trainer with a deep laceration to his thigh. The cut is approximately 1/8 inch deep, 1 inch long, and bleeding moderately. What would be the proper steps for the athletic trainer to take to treat this wound?
     A. Use a pressure bandage to control the bleeding, keep the wound clean and free of debris, use steri-strips for temporary closure, and apply ice and compression to the area
     B. Use a pressure bandage to control the bleeding, keep the wound clean, suture the laceration, and cover with a sterile dressing
     C. Wipe the area clean with soap and water, use an antibiotic ointment to minimize infection, suture the wound, and cover it with a sterile dressing
     D. Wipe the area clean with soap and water, apply a large adhesive band-aid, and apply ice to the area

114. An athlete comes to the athletic trainer holding a tooth that has just been knocked out of his mouth. What would be the proper steps for the athletic trainer to take to allow for a successful reimplantation?
     A. Try to put it back in place and use a topical ointment for pain
     B. Put the tooth in a jar of water, tell the athlete to store it in a refrigerator until he can see a dentist
     C. There is nothing the athletic trainer can do because the tooth is dead
     D. Place the tooth in a cloth soaked with saline or water and get the athlete to a dentist within 30 minutes

115. During an emergency, all of the following information should be given over the telephone by the athletic trainer to emergency personnel **except**:
     A. The type of emergency
     B. The current status of the athlete
     C. The name of the next of kin
     D. The type of treatment currently being given to the athlete

116. An athlete has a suspected fracture involving the knee. Which of the following areas should be splinted?
    A. The ankle and lower leg areas
    B. The knee and thigh
    C. The ankle, knee, and thigh
    D. The lower limb joints and one side of the trunk

117. Under what condition(s) is an athlete likely to experience a stress fracture of a bone?
    A. After a few high loads or many small loads are applied to the bone
    B. After a large traumatic insult to the bone
    C. After a traumatic incident which is quickly followed by a few small loads to the bone
    D. After one or two small loads are applied to the bone

Rehabilitation of Athletic Injuries

1. Which muscle grade denotes active muscle movement in a gravity-eliminated position?
    A. -3/5
    B. 3+/5
    C. 2/5
    D. 1/5

2. All of the following tests are useful in evaluating low back pathology **except**:
    A. Valsalva's maneuver
    B. Bilateral straight leg test
    C. Scouring test
    D. Lasegue test

3. What does an "extension lag" mean?
    A. Ability to only flex the knee
    B. Inability to fully backward bend (lumbar movement)
    C. One leg drags behind the other during gait
    D. Inability to fully extend the knee

4. What is the best method of determining the recovery status of the hand and forearm after injury?
    A. Use of a KT-1000 arthrometer
    B. Assessing the strength of a handshake
    C. Manual muscle testing of the wrist
    D. Use of a hand dynamometer

5. What is the best position for the athlete to be in to muscle test the piriformis?
    A. Sitting
    B. Prone
    C. Supine
    D. Sidelying

6. What is the average range of motion of elbow flexion?
    A. 0° to 90°
    B. 0° to 135°
    C. 0° to 115°
    D. 0° to 100°

7.   What is the proper method to manually muscle test the biceps femoris muscle?
     A. Sitting, resisting knee extension
     B. Lying prone, resisting knee flexion with the tibia in external rotation
     C. Sitting, resisting hip flexion
     D. Lying prone, resisting knee flexion with the tibia in internal rotation

8.   What is a quick method of testing the motor ability of the S1 nerve root?
     A. Have the athlete walk on his or her toes
     B. Manually resist ankle inversion
     C. Manually resist great toe extension
     D. Assess the athlete's ability to squat

9.   To test the function of the rhomboid major muscle, the athletic trainer should ask the athlete to perform what movement?
     A. Scapular retraction
     B. Shoulder internal rotation
     C. Scapular protraction
     D. Shoulder shrug

10. Which muscle supinates the forearm and flexes the shoulder?
     A. Brachialis
     B. Coracobrachialis
     C. Biceps brachii
     D. Flexor pollicis longus

11. All of the following movements occur in the sagittal plane **except**:
     A. Hip abduction
     B. Shoulder flexion
     C. Knee extension
     D. Hip flexion

12. Which muscle flexes both the foot and the knee?
     A. Biceps femoris
     B. Flexor digitorum
     C. Posterior tibialis
     D. Gastrocnemius

13. The flexor pollicis longus is responsible for which of the following action(s):
     A. Great toe flexion
     B. Thumb flexion
     C. Thumb flexion and adduction
     D. Thumb flexion and abduction

14. Asking the athlete to move his or her eyes from side to side and up and down tests the integrity of which cranial nerve?
     A. II
     B. V
     C. I
     D. III

15. The rectus femoris muscle _____ and _____ when it contracts.
    A. Flexes the hip, externally rotates the hip
    B. Extends the hip, flexes the knee
    C. Flexes the knee, plantar flexes the ankle
    D. Flexes the hip, extends the knee

16. Which of the following muscles is **not** involved in internal rotation of the hip?
    A. Adductor magnus
    B. Gluteus maximus
    C. Gracilis
    D. Tensor fascia latae

17. Which of the cervical nerve roots below represent the sensory dermatomes of the hand?
    I.   C5   IV. C8
    II. C6   V. T1
    III. C7

    A. I, II, III
    B. II, III IV
    C. III, IV, V
    D. I, III, IV

18. Which of the following muscles does **not** adduct the shoulder?
    A. Pectoralis major
    B. Teres major
    C. Subscapularis
    D. Serratus anterior

19. Which of the following muscles does **not** extend the trunk?
    A. Semispinalis (thoracic)
    B. Erector spinae
    C. Quadratus lumborum
    D. Multifidi

20. The supinator muscle is innervated by which of the following nerves?
    A. Musculocutaneous nerve
    B. Axillary nerve
    C. Radial nerve
    D. Median nerve

21. Following multiple ankle sprains over the course of the year, the athletic trainer detects some weakness of the invertors and evertors of an athlete's ankle. Which of the following muscles does **not** invert the ankle?
    A. Tibialis posterior
    B. Extensor digitorum longus
    C. Flexor digitorum longus
    D. Flexor hallucis longus

22. During digestion, food passes through the small intestine as it is being broken down into smaller components. Of the following, which area of the small intestine does it pass through first?
    A. Ileum
    B. Duodenum
    C. Jejunum
    D. Cecum

23. What nerve passes through the carpal tunnel?
    A. Musculocutaneous
    B. Radial
    C. Median
    D. Ulnar

24. All of the following bones make up the pelvis **except**:
    A. Coccyx
    B. Sacrum
    C. Ileum
    D. Innominate bones

25. Which nerves innervate the hip adductor musculature?
    A. Femoral, superior gluteal
    B. Femoral, tibial
    C. Femoral, obturator
    D. Femoral, obturator, inferior gluteal

26. Which of the following muscles abducts the little finger of the hand?
    A. Interossei
    B. Abductor digiti minimi
    C. Lumbricals
    D. Abductor digitorum brevis

27. Which of the following muscles does **not** extend and laterally flex the neck?
    A. Splenius capitis
    B. Splenius cervicis
    C. Levator scapulae
    D. Sternocleidomastoid

28. Which of these muscles are innervated by the tibial nerve?
    I.   Gastrocnemius   IV. Tibialis anterior
    II. Flexor hallucis longus V. Biceps femoris
    III. Extensor hallucis longus

    A. I, II, III, IV
    B. II, III, V
    C. I, II, V
    D. I, III, IV, V

29. All of the following are controlled by the cranial nerves **except**:
    A. Vision
    B. Olfactory
    C. Tongue movement
    D. Cervical flexion

30. Which of the following is the correct sequence of tissue healing?
    A. Cellular response, regeneration, remodeling
    B. Remodeling, regeneration, cellular response
    C. Rejection, regeneration, resolution
    D. Regeneration, resolution, remodeling

31. Which of the following cells release histamine and serotonin during the cellular response phase of tissue healing?
    A. Macrophages
    B. Mast cells and platelets
    C. Granulocytes
    D. Leukocytes

32. What amount of time may it take for complete remodeling of tissues to occur after a soft tissue injury?
    A. 1 to 3 months
    B. 6 to 9 months
    C. Up to 1 year
    D. 12 to 24 months

33. Where is the primary location for ATP production in skeletal muscle?
    A. Sarcomere
    B. Sarcoplasm
    C. Sarcolemma
    D. Sarcoplasmic reticulum

34. Sensory receptors located at the musculotendinous junction, which monitor active tension generated by the muscle during a contraction, are called:
    A. Pacinian corpuscles
    B. Ruffinian receptors
    C. Golgi tendon organs
    D. Muscle spindles

35. The acute phase of an injury lasts approximately 3 to 4 days. What occurs at the time of initial trauma?
    A. Phagocytosis, followed by vasoconstriction and diapedesis
    B. Transitory vasodilatation, inflammation, and phagocytosis
    C. Transitory vasoconstriction, followed by vasodilatation and increased permeability
    D. Vasoconstriction, increased permeability, and granulation

36. Which of the following describes a neurapraxia?
    A. Demyelination of the axon sheath that leads to a conduction block. Usually heals in approximately 1 to 2 weeks.
    B. Loss or disruption of the axon and myelin sheath. The epineurium is still intact.
    C. An injury to the endoneurium, perineurium, and epineurium with a permanent neurological deficit.
    D. A crush injury to a nerve causing damage to the epineurium. The perineurium is intact.

37. Bone grows via a process of apposition and resorption on its surface. Which of the following cells are responsible for the resorption of bone during its growth or repair?
    A. Osteoblasts
    B. Osteocytes
    C. Osteophils
    D. Osteoclasts

38. Why is the repair response so limited in the articular cartilage of a joint after an injury in the adult athlete?
    A. Articular cartilage cells do not undergo mitosis in the mature athlete
    B. Articular cartilage has a poor venous supply
    C. Articular cartilage has a low water content
    D. There are fewer mitochondria present in articular cartilage than in hyaline cartilage

39. Where do primitive stem cells mature into mature red and white blood cells and platelets?
    A. Liver
    B. Spleen
    C. Gallbladder
    D. None of the above

40. What are the four sensations an athlete will experience with the application of cryotherapy?
    A. Cold, burning, cramping, numbness
    B. Pain, aching, stinging, cold
    C. Aching, burning, pain, numbness
    D. Cold, burning, aching, numbness

41. The effects of treating a subacute musculoskeletal injury with a warm whirlpool include all of the following **except**:
    A. Analgesia
    B. Stimulation of local circulation
    C. Decrease muscle spasm
    D. Increase deep tissue temperature

42. Which cells are active after an injury to begin building collagen?
    A. Fibroblasts
    B. Osteoblasts
    C. Granulocytes
    D. Osteoclasts

43. Heat is dissipated in the body by all of the following means **except**:
    A. Shivering
    B. Convection
    C. The lungs
    D. Sweat evaporation

44. External muscular force available for useful work is the result of all of the following factors **except**:
    A. The velocity of muscular shortening
    B. Whether the muscle is fast or slow twitch
    C. The angle of the pull of the muscle
    D. The length of the muscle

45. Balance and coordination are critical for athletic performance. Feedback from the muscles as to what they are doing during a particular activity is known as _____. The area of the brain that assists in controlling movement is the _____.
    A. Proprioception, brain stem
    B. Muscle perception, medulla
    C. Kinesthesia, cortex
    D. Proprioception, cerebellum

46. A stretching exercise that consists of a "stretch and hold" position is known as:
    A. Static stretch
    B. PNF pattern
    C. Ballistic stretch
    D. Warm-up

47. During aerobic exercise, if hyperventilation does **not** adequately increase the oxygen supply in the blood, what must occur to meet the gas exchange demands?
    A. Increased cardiac output
    B. Decreased cardiac output
    C. Supplemental iron pills must be provided
    D. The activity must be discontinued

48. An athlete has just been injured on the basketball court, and the athletic trainer begins administering first aid. During the initial contact, the trainer notices the athlete is hyperactive, argumentative, and is sarcastic in his responses to questions. All of the following actions by the athletic trainer are inappropriate **except**:
    A. Telling the athlete he is not acting appropriately
    B. Being abrupt and telling the athlete to snap out of it
    C. Allowing the athlete to express his emotions as they occur
    D. Calling the coach over to calm the athlete

49. An injured athlete is led through a therapeutic mental process in which he pictures himself being evaluated by the athletic trainer and assured the injury is not serious; then he pictures himself moving through rehabilitation and recovering nicely, and finally, returning to his sport fully healed. This therapeutic approach to the recovery process is known as:
    A. Regression
    B. Thought stopping
    C. Visualization
    D. Meditation

50. In order for the rehabilitation of an injured athlete to be successful, what must the athletic trainer establish with the athlete prior to and during the rehabilitation?
    A. A good rapport
    B. A position of dominance
    C. A deadline by which the athlete must return to full-time participation in his or her sport
    D. That the coach has the final decision in his or her rehabilitation sessions

51. A basketball player who has sprained her ankle for the second time in 3 months reports to the athletic training room for her third treatment session. The athletic trainer notices she is demanding and wants to know why the athletic trainer "did not fix her ankle the right way the first time." She becomes somewhat threatening, stating that she will find someone else to help her if she is not successfully helped this time. The best response to an attention-seeking athlete by the athletic trainer would be:
    A. Give up and let her seek help elsewhere
    B. Work with the athlete as long as necessary to satisfy her need for attention
    C. Set specific but reasonable time limits with the athlete per treatment session so the athletic trainer is not overtaxed
    D. Encourage the athlete to take a more positive position on her rehabilitation and use humor to divert her attention away from the injury

52. The athletic trainer notices an athlete is prone to abnormal bruising. After discussing the problem with the team MD, the doctor recommends which of the following vitamins?
    A. Vitamin E
    B. Vitamin D
    C. Vitamin K
    D. Niacin

53. If an athlete needs to lose weight for health reasons, how many calories must his or her daily diet be reduced by in order to lose 1 to 2 pounds per week?
    A. 250 to 500 calories/day
    B. 1000 to 2000 calories/week
    C. 1000 to 2000 calories/day
    D. 500 to 1000 calories/day

54. If the desired therapeutic effect is decreased pain, edema, and inflammation, which modality would be best utilized?
    A. Moist heat packs
    B. Ultrasound
    C. Ice packs
    D. Fluidotherapy

55. Heat-producing currents in the body that are formed by a magnetic field that is externally applied in short-wave diathermy are called:
    A. Induction currents
    B. Magnetic currents
    C. Eddy currents
    D. Alternating currents

56. High-voltage pulsed monophasic generators (HVPG) deliver current to deep tissues without damaging superficial tissues and are used for pain modulation. What type of waveform is used with this type of stimulator?
    A. Asymmetrical, biphasic spiked pulse
    B. Monophasic squared pulse
    C. Symmetrical biphasic pulses
    D. Monophasic spike delivered in pairs

57. A moist heat pack causes all the following effects **except**:
    A. Higher superficial tissue temperatures
    B. Increases in muscle tissue temperatures
    C. Sedation
    D. Reduction of muscle spasms

58. What physiological effects occur under the cathode of an electrical stimulator?
    I.   Vasodilatation
    II. Vasoconstriction
    III. Tissue softening
    IV. Irritation

    A. I, III, IV
    B. II, III, IV
    C. I, II, III
    D. I, II, IV

59. All of the following are contraindications for using cryotherapy **except**:
    A. Raynaud's phenomenon
    B. Inflammation
    C. Vasculitis
    D. Cold urticaria

60. A functional skill for an athlete in an ankle rehabilitation program would be:
    A. Gastrocnemius flexibility
    B. Single-leg hopping
    C. Lifting tolerance
    D. Anterior tibialis strength

61. When rehabilitating a musculoskeletal injury, what is the proper progression of treatment?
    A. Range of motion, strength, endurance, proprioception
    B. Pain relief, agility, range of motion, strength
    C. Range of motion, pain relief, endurance, proprioception
    D. Proprioception, range of motion, strength, endurance

62. Which of the following PNF techniques is **not** a strengthening technique?
    A. Slow reversal
    B. Rhythmic stabilization
    C. Slow-reversal-hold-relax
    D. Rhythmic initiation

63. During a lower extremity D1 flexion PNF pattern, what movements are taking place at the hip?
    A. Extension, abduction, internal rotation
    B. Flexion, abduction, internal rotation
    C. Extension, adduction, external rotation
    D. Flexion, adduction, external rotation

64. During a D2 extension pattern of the upper extremity, what is the proper timing sequence?
    A. Shoulder extension, forearm pronation, finger flexion
    B. Shoulder flexion, scapular retraction, finger extension
    C. Shoulder abduction, forearm supination, finger extension
    D. Shoulder extension, forearm supination, finger flexion

65. According to Maitland's five grades of joint motion, which grade would be most appropriate when joint movement is limited by pain and spasm?
    A. I
    B. II
    C. III
    D. IV

66. An athlete is seen by the athletic trainer 4 weeks postoperatively after shoulder arthroscopy. During the athletic trainer's assessment, it is found the athlete has limited abduction secondary to capsular stiffness. Which of the following joint glides would be appropriate to improve this motion?
    A. Inferior humeral glide
    B. Anterior humeral glide
    C. Posterior humeral glide
    D. Superior humeral glide

67. Which of the following statements accurately describes isokinetic training?
    A. Generation of a muscular force with no viable joint movement
    B. Generation of a muscular force with visible joint movement that occurs at a constant speed but with variable external resistance
    C. Generation of a muscular force with visible joint movement at a variable speed but with a fixed external resistance
    D. Generation of a muscle force during muscular lengthening

68. Which of the following massage techniques are methods of tapotement?
    A. Cupping
    B. Hacking
    C. Pinching
    D. All of the above

69. When massage is utilized to induce a sedative effect, which type of massage technique is indicated?
    A. Tapotement
    B. Vibration
    C. Petrissage
    D. Effleurage

70. What conditioning component is needed to perceive the position of the foot as it lands on the ground after the swing phase of gait?
    A. Agility
    B. Balance
    C. Proprioception
    D. Kinesthesia

71. Descending hills during running requires what type of muscular contraction by the quadriceps to decelerate the body?
    A. Positive
    B. Concentric
    C. Isokinetic
    D. Eccentric

72. What should a post-season conditioning program specifically focus on?
    A. Endurance activities
    B. Strengthening and flexibility exercises
    C. Sport-specific activities
    D. Identifying and improving the areas of conditioning that the athlete is deficient in

73. During the acute phase of an ankle injury, the water temperature of a whirlpool should be set at what temperature?
    A. 37° to 37.7° C
    B. 55° to 65° F
    C. 30° to 35° F
    D. 70° to 80° F

74. Before returning an athlete to full activity, all of the following criteria should equal those taken from the uninvolved side at the end of the rehabilitation program **except**:
    A. Strength of each muscle group
    B. Girth measurements at 6 inches above and below the joint line
    C. Proprioception of both extremities
    D. Flexibility of the involved muscle groups

75. Which of the following components of a rehabilitation program is most often overlooked by the athletic trainer during rehabilitation?
    A. Endurance
    B. Flexibility
    C. Proprioception
    D. Functional testing prior to return to the sport

76. What type of exercises may be safely initiated immediately after knee surgery?
    A. Closed-chain eccentric exercises
    B. Isotonic exercises
    C. Isometric exercises
    D. Functional exercises

77. When rehabilitating an athlete who has been diagnosed with "jumper's knee," which muscle group should eventually be strengthened?
    A. Hamstrings
    B. Quadriceps
    C. Hip adductors
    D. Hip extensors

78. When treating an athlete with trochanteric bursitis, flexibility should be increased in which of the following muscles?
    A. Gluteus maximus
    B. Tensor fascia latae
    C. Iliacus
    D. Piriformis

79. A tight Achilles' tendon can cause _____ or _____ in order to allow the lower leg to move over the foot during running.
    A. Late heel-off, early heel strike
    B. Early heel-off, excessive supination
    C. Late heel-off, late toe-off
    D. Early heel-off, excessive pronation

80. Which of the following is **not** a factor in designing an appropriate treatment program?
    A. The stage of tissue healing
    B. Pain with joint motion
    C. The severity of the injury
    D. How soon the coach feels the athlete should return to play

81. When rehabilitating a cervical strain, the athletic trainer must also maintain the integrity of the:
    A. Shoulder girdle
    B. Upper back
    C. Upper arm
    D. Hand

82. Which of the following sequences are appropriate steps in rehabilitating a grade II ankle sprain?
    A. RICE, stretching the Achilles' tendon, isometric exercises, proprioceptive exercises, followed by isotonic exercises
    B. RICE, isotonic exercises, hopping exercises, stretching the Achilles' tendon, active range-of-motion exercises
    C. RICE, isotonic exercises, followed by isokinetic exercises, active range of motion exercises
    D. RICE, treadmill ambulation, active range of motion exercises, figure-eight exercises, stretching of the Achilles' tendon, foot intrinsic exercises

83. What is the best time to begin a rehabilitation program after an injury?
    A. Immediately
    B. After the injured part is "healed"
    C. After the inflammation is under control
    D. Once the pain subsides

84. When following the DAPRE technique of progressive resistive exercise, the first set of 10 repetitions is performed with a weight that is _____ of the weight that will be lifted in set three.
    A. 50%
    B. 25%
    C. 100%
    D. 75%

85. When rehabilitating an athlete with patellofemoral pain syndrome, which muscle groups should be strengthened?
    A. Quadriceps, hamstrings
    B. Hip abductors, hamstrings
    C. Hip adductors, quadriceps
    D. Hip flexors, hip external rotators

86. Which of the following exercises are appropriate in attempting to decrease the symptoms of thoracic outlet syndrome?
    A. Cervical range of motion exercises, anterior shoulder strengthening
    B. Cervical range of motion exercises, cervical isometrics
    C. Anterior chest wall strengthening, cervical isometrics
    D. Stretching the anterior chest wall, strengthening the posterior mid-thoracic area

87. What are the most appropriate exercises for a diagnosis of lumbar spinal stenosis?
    A. Williams' flexion exercises
    B. McKenzie extension exercises
    C. Lumbar stabilization exercises
    D. Postural awareness exercises

88. Which of the following exercises does **not** address proprioception?
    A. Recumbent stationary bicycling
    B. Mini-tramp exercises
    C. Stork-standing exercises with the eyes open
    D. Treadmill exercises

89. When rehabilitating a shoulder, where is the first area strengthening exercises should be initiated?
    A. Rotator cuff musculature
    B. Cervical musculature
    C. Scapular musculature
    D. Shoulder abductors, flexors, and internal rotators

90. When rehabilitating an athlete who has undergone an anterior cruciate ligament reconstruction, which of the following muscle groups must be strengthened to support the graft?
    A. Triceps surae
    B. Hip adductors
    C. Quadriceps
    D. Hamstrings

91. Which of the following pieces of equipment is **not** considered closed chain?
    A. Treadmill
    B. Leg-press machine
    C. Upper body ergometer
    D. Isokinetic knee extension machine

92. When rehabilitating tennis elbow, which muscular group should be strengthened?
    A. Wrist flexors
    B. Wrist extensors
    C. Elbow flexors
    D. Elbow extensors

93. When rehabilitating an athlete with a recent herniated lumbar disc, which of the following exercises are most appropriate?
    A. Williams' flexion exercises
    B. McKenzie extension exercises
    C. Lumbar stabilization exercises
    D. Posterior pelvic tilts and knee to chest exercises

94. An athlete needs instruction on how to properly perform an abdominal sit-up. What should the athletic trainer recommend to him?
    A. Place his hands behind his head, take a deep breath and hold it, and pull his torso up toward his bent knees
    B. Cross his arms across his chest, tuck in his chin, bend his knees up, inhale and then exhale as he pulls his torso up toward his knees
    C. Place his hands behind his head, bend his knees, exhale completely first, and inhale deeply as he pulls his torso up toward his knees
    D. Keeping his arms down by his sides, bend up his knees, inhale deeply and hold it as he pulls his torso up toward his knees

95. Knee braces can be classified as either functional, prophylactic, or rehabilitative. Which type of brace would likely be worn for 1 to 2 weeks after a grade II medial collateral ligament tear?
    A. Functional
    B. Prophylactic
    C. Rehabilitative
    D. No brace is necessary for this injury

96. In terms of specificity of training, which type of exercise would be appropriate during the late phases of rehabilitation of a soccer player?
    A. Stairmaster
    B. Swimming
    C. Stationary bicycling
    D. Treadmill exercise

97. Which of the following conditions is **not** indicated for mechanical traction?
    A. Interspinous sprains
    B. Degenerative joint disease
    C. Herniated discs or protrusions
    D. Degenerative disc disease

98. Which of the muscle groups below are involved during a bench press?
    - I.   Anterior deltoid
    - II. Rhomboids
    - III. Triceps
    - IV. Pectoralis major
    - V.   Latissimus dorsi
    - VI. Upper trapezius

    - A. I, II, III, IV
    - B. III, IV, V, VI
    - C. I, III, IV, V
    - D. II, III, IV, VI

99. Which of the following muscle groups are involved during a full squat with weights?
    - I.   Quadriceps
    - II. Hamstrings
    - III. Erector spinae
    - IV. Middle deltoid
    - V.   Gluteus maximus
    - VI. Serratus anterior

    - A. I, II, IV, V
    - B. II, III, IV, V
    - C. I, II, III, V
    - D. II, III, V, VI

100. Which of the following muscles are involved in a seated military press?
    - I.   Trapezius
    - II. Latissimus dorsi
    - III. Pectoralis major
    - IV. Serratus anterior
    - V.   Posterior deltoid
    - VI. Triceps

    - A. II, III, VI
    - B. I, III, IV, V
    - C. I, IV, V, VI
    - D. I, III, IV, VI

101. Which of the following describes a grade III joint mobilization technique?
    - A. Small amplitude movement at the end range
    - B. Large amplitude movement throughout the full available range of motion of the joint
    - C. Small amplitude movement in the beginning of the range of motion
    - D. Thrusting movement done at the anatomical limits of the joint

102. When rehabilitating an athlete, it is important that the area being rehabilitated is stressed with a variety of intensities and durations during conditioning. The body responds to these stresses by adapting to the specific demands imposed on it. What is this principle known as?
    - A. The SAID principle
    - B. The DAPRE principle
    - C. The RICE principle
    - D. The SITS principle

103. Which of the following is **not** an example of an isotonic device?
    - A. Free weights
    - B. A nautilus machine
    - C. A wall
    - D. Wall pulleys

104. When stretching during a warm-up routine, which type of stretching should **not** be encouraged because it may lead to an injury?
    A. Ballistic
    B. Active
    C. Static
    D. Plyometric

105. In which of the following sports would plyometric training be beneficial?
    A. Rock climbing
    B. Cross-country
    C. Volleyball
    D. Archery

106. Which of the following exercises improves proprioceptive feedback when rehabilitating a lower extremity injury?
    A. Stationary bicycling
    B. Single-leg standing on a mini-tramp
    C. Using a knee extension machine
    D. Bilateral calf raises

107. An athlete is recovering from a partial meniscectomy performed 1 week ago. All of the following actions would be appropriate at this time **except**:
    A. Achilles' stretching
    B. Four quadrant straight leg raises
    C. Stationary bicycling with minimal/no resistance
    D. Eccentric quadriceps strengthening

108. Which of the following exercises should be avoided in the early stages (phase I) of anterior cruciate reconstruction rehabilitation?
    A. Full knee extension exercise
    B. Resisted hip abduction
    C. Toe raises
    D. Hamstring curls

109. Two exercises that are designed to stabilize the lumbar spine during low back rehabilitation include _____ and _____.
    A. Single knee to chest exercise, double knee to chest
    B. Hamstring stretching, bridging exercises
    C. Partial sit-ups, active trunk extension in prone
    D. Resisted hip abduction exercise, iliotibial band stretching

110. An athletic trainer working in a sports medicine clinic may have to read a SOAP note. In what section would a finding such as a positive Lachman's test be recorded?
    A. Subjective (S)
    B. Objective (O)
    C. Assessment (A)
    D. Plan (P)

Health Care Administration

1. The athletic trainer of a collegiate women's swimming and diving team suspects one of his athlete's might have a severe eating disorder. After lengthy discussions with both the coach and athlete, the athletic trainer decides it would be best for the athlete if she is referred for professional help. To which of the following professionals should the athlete be referred?
   A. An endocrinologist
   B. A psychologist
   C. A registered dietitian
   D. A registered nurse

2. All of the following forms are a critical part of the athlete's permanent medical record and should be completed before the athlete is permitted to participate in the first team practice **except**:
   A. Permission-to-treat form
   B. Preseason physical form
   C. Release form for athletes subjected to high risk
   D. Coach's injury report form

3. A policy can be defined as:
   A. A specific plan for members of an organization to follow
   B. A broad statement of an intended action
   C. An organizational plan that provides program direction for 1 or 2 years
   D. A mission statement of an organization

4. The floor of an athletic training room can be comprised of all the following materials **except**:
   A. Vinyl
   B. Wood
   C. Concrete
   D. Rubber

5. Which of the following should be included in a preparticipation physical?
   I.   Height and weight   IV. Ear/nose/throat exam
   II. Orthopedic screening   V. Blood work
   III. Vital signs

   A. I, II, V
   B. II, IV, V
   C. I, II III, IV
   D. I, III, V

6. Maintaining up-to-date records is extremely important. The athletic trainer should document how often?
   A. Monthly
   B. Weekly
   C. Daily
   D. Every 6 months

7. An athletic trainer can release an athlete's medical records to which of the following?
    A. Professional athletic team organizations
    B. Insurance companies
    C. The media
    D. No organization or individual without the consent of the athlete or a legal guardian

8. A high school athlete is pitching during a baseball game and is hit in the head with a line drive. He is seriously injured. The assistant coach is also the athlete's father. In this situation, who is legally responsible for the athlete's immediate care?
    A. The head coach
    B. The assistant coach/parent
    C. The athletic trainer
    D. The high school at which the event is taking place

9. Athletic trainers should carry what type of insurance?
    A. Catastrophic event insurance
    B. Professional liability insurance
    C. Accident insurance
    D. Life insurance

10. _____ charting is a form of record keeping that allows the athletic trainer to list the athlete's injury information, the actions taken by the athletic trainer, and the response of the athlete to the athletic trainer's treatment in column form.
    A. SOAP notes
    B. Focus charting
    C. Charting by exception
    D. Computerized documentation

11. You have been given the opportunity to assist in hiring a new team physician. What type of agreement should be drawn up between the school and the physician?
    A. School emergency systems agreement
    B. A noncompete agreement
    C. A medical consent agreement
    D. A physician's letter of agreement

12. Which of the following models of supervision for a head athletic trainer could be described as a "mentoring" approach?
    A. Developmental supervision
    B. Inspection supervision
    C. On-field supervision
    D. Clinical supervision

13. You have been asked to initiate a student athletic training program in your high school. One of the areas you are covering is "sexually transmitted diseases." The following topics relating to AIDS should include all of the following **except**:
    A. Blood-borne pathogens
    B. HIV testing
    C. Universal precautions
    D. Bacterial infections

14. Which of the following best describes an athletic trainer in a nontraditional athletic training setting?
    A. Manager
    B. Organizer
    C. Director
    D. Planner

15. You are employed at a local high school as an athletic trainer and have been asked by your principal to refer any ill students to your school nurse. Who is responsible for the care of the student athletes in this situation?
    A. School nurse
    B. School physician
    C. Athletic trainer
    D. School principal

16. What guidelines does the athletic trainer have to follow regarding maintaining proper hygiene and sanitation in the athletic training room?
    A. Joint Commission on Accreditation of Healthcare Organizations (JCAHO)
    B. American Medical Association (AMA)
    C. Rehabilitation Accreditation Commission (CARF)
    D. Occupational Safety and Health Administration (OSHA)

17. Which of the following organizations establishes standards of quality for organizations that provide rehabilitative services?
    A. Joint Commission on Accreditation of Healthcare Organizations (JCAHO)
    B. American Medical Association (AMA)
    C. Commision on Accreditation of Rehabilitation Facilities (CARF)
    D. Occupational Safety and Health Administration (OSHA)

18. All of the following are components of a well-written SOAP note **except**:
    A. It is legible, clear, and concise
    B. It contains many objective measurements
    C. Progress is expressed in functional terms
    D. It is written with the intent to mislead an insurance company

19. Which of the following documents would be most likely to be subpoenaed during a civil litigation suit against an athletic trainer?
    A. Equipment inventory
    B. Treatment log
    C. Budget reports
    D. Sporting event schedules

20. Fixed payments made on a monthly basis to a managed care provider is known as what type of reimbursement?
    A. Point-of-service plan
    B. Fee for service
    C. Third-party reimbursement
    D. Capitation

21. Which of the following can cause an indirect sports fatality?
     A. Contact sports
     B. A blow to the head
     C. Heatstroke
     D. Rodeo riding

22. One of your athletes has just purchased a bicycle helmet and found a crack in the shell. To which
     organization should the manufacturer of the helmet report this defect?
     A. National Athletic Trainers' Association (NATA)
     B. Consumer Product Safety Commission
     C. National Operating Committee for Athletic Equipment
     D. United States Olympic Committee (USOC)

23. Which of the following forms should the athletic trainer fill out to gain the quickest reimbursement
     from an insurance company?
     A. HCFA -1500 form
     B. CPT 1 -A form
     C. UCR form
     D. An incident report form

24. The athletic trainer may use any of the following to treat an injured or ill athlete **except:**
     A. A prescription drug
     B. Hydrotherapy
     C. Cryotherapy
     D. Electrotherapy

25. Maintaining accurate medical records is the responsibility of which of the following individuals in the
     high school setting:
     I.   Athletic trainer   IV. School nurse
     II. Athletic director   V.   Team physician
     III. Principal

     A. I, II, III
     B. II, IV, V
     C. III, IV, V
     D. I, IV, V

26. During a pre-participation examination, what type of assessment should be utilized to document the
     maturity of an athlete's secondary sexual characteristics?
     A. Tanner's five stages of assessment
     B. HOPS assessment scale
     C. Glasgow scale
     D. Erickson's hierarchy

27. An athletic trainer discovers that he is infected with the HIV virus. All of the following would be prudent steps for the trainer to take **except**:
    A. Avoid seeking medical care
    B. Inform, if or when it becomes appropriate to do so, his patients, coworkers, or supervisors of his status
    C. Take the necessary steps to avoid the possibility of infecting others
    D. Make sure he has ongoing medical evaluations

28. What type of analysis would be considered a useful tool in the strategic planning of an existing athletic training program?
    A. The HICFA analysis
    B. The strengths/weaknesses analysis
    C. The WOTS-UP analysis
    D. The Samson analysis

29. The statute of limitations involving a negligence suit has a limit of how many years?
    A. Up to 2 years
    B. 1 to 3 years
    C. 7 to 10 years
    D. 10 to 15 years

30. The primary care physician who is appointed by an insurance company to oversee the medical care given to an athlete and assigns any specialty and ancillary services is referred to as:
    A. The gatekeeper
    B. The participating provider
    C. The third-party administrator
    D. The policy holder

31. The _____ is a charge that represents the maximum amount that an insurance company will pay a provider.
    A. UCR
    B. NCR
    C. ADA
    D. CPT

32. Which type of insurance should the athletic trainer carry in case of a criminal complaint involving negligence?
    A. General secondary insurance
    B. Catastrophic insurance
    C. Accident insurance
    D. Professional liability insurance

33. An athlete and his coach from your wrestling program have been trying to convince you that the athlete, who has been diagnosed with impetigo, can return early to wrestle. Your response should be based upon which NATA Code of Ethics principle?
    A. Principle I
    B. Principle II
    C. Principle III
    D. Principle V

34. The _____ is a nongovernmental, nonprofit organization that gathers injury data from a number of sources including educational institutions.
    A. National Safety Council
    B. NOCSAE
    C. ACSM
    D. OSHA

35. Which organization must certify face masks that are used in ice hockey helmets?
    A. Canadian Standard Association (CSA)
    B. Hockey Equipment Certification Council (HECC)
    C. National Operating Committee on Standards for Athletic Equipment
    D. American Society for Testing Material (ASTM)

36. All of the following are types of state regulation status for athletic trainers **except**:
    I.   Certification   IV. Registration
    II. Licensing   V. Inactive
    III. Active

    A. I, II, V
    B. II, III, IV
    C. I, II, IV
    D. II, IV, V

37. _____ supplies include such items as adhesive tape, gauze pads, and band-aids.
    A. Expendable
    B. Capital
    C. Nonexpendable
    D. Nonfixed

38. _____, _____, and _____ must be taken into consideration when developing a risk management plan.
    A. Security, liability, competence
    B. Security, fire safety, and management of emergency injuries
    C. Insurance procedures, policies/procedures, materials
    D. Licensing, certifications, administrative policy

39. During a pre-participation examination, the team physician and athletic trainer should **jointly**:
    A. Perform blood tests
    B. Perform a Snellen test
    C. Review each examination for the final approval to participate
    D. Perform an orthopedic screening

40. Who should make the final decision regarding if an athlete with a disability can participate in a sport according to the Americans with Disabilities Act?
    A. Athletic trainer
    B. Team physician
    C. Individual athlete
    D. Parents

41. Large purchases for an educational institution are usually done through a process known as:
    A. Direct purchase
    B. Indirect purchase
    C. Soliciting
    D. Bid process

42. All of the following are steps an athletic trainer can take to avoid litigation **except**:
    A. Develop a comprehensive emergency plan
    B. Establish a detailed, written job description
    C. Establish a yearly plan for modality maintainance
    D. Keep accurate records of all prescription medication dispensed

43. Which of the following best describes what a "copayment" is?
    A. An occasional payment made by a policy holder to an insurance company
    B. The amount owed yearly by the policy holder before the insurance company will begin to pay for services
    C. The amount of money that both an employee and employer share when paying for medical benefits
    D. A percentage of the total amount the policy holder is required to pay for medical services rendered

44. An athletic trainer is working in a clinical setting. Which of the following populations is the athletic trainer best suited to treat?
    A. Neurologically impaired
    B. Physically active
    C. Burn patients
    D. Geriatric patients

45. You are in the position to hire an assistant athletic trainer. You have a specific person in mind but your athletic director implies he is not comfortable with this person's gender. Which level of the law mandates the hiring and firing of employees?
    A. State
    B. Local
    C. Federal
    D. District

Professional Development and Responsibility

1. Which of the following individuals are most susceptible to heatstroke, and therefore must be carefully educated regarding the importance of adequate fluid intake during activity in hot, humid weather?
   A. Basketball guard
   B. Defensive lineman in football
   C. Female gymnast
   D. Swimmer

2. When using an ice pack to decrease pain and swelling of an injured limb at home, what should the athletic trainer recommend to the athlete to prevent a cryotherapy injury?
   A. Add acetone to the ice at a 3:1 ratio
   B. Keep the injured limb elevated while using ice
   C. Place a damp towel between the athlete's skin and the ice pack
   D. Leave the ice pack on the body part between 20 to 40 minutes at a time

3.   One of your athletes has been diagnosed with impetigo. What should the athletic trainer recommed to the athlete to prevent spread of the infection to other individuals?
      A. Clean his clothing daily with bleach
      B. Wear gloves
      C. Practice safe sex
      D. Prevent others from borrowing his clothing or use his towels

4.   One of your male athletes notices a tingling sensation in his urethra followed by a discharge of greenish yellow pus from his penis. He is also complaining of pain during urination. You suspect which sexually transmitted disease and recommend which of the following actions?
      A. Syphilis; have the athlete take Zovirax for a week to 10 days
      B. Trichomoniasis; have the athlete drink acidic fluids, call his family physician, and have the athlete refrain from all sexual contact
      C. Genital candidiasis; have the athlete apply a fungicide to his penis
      D. Gonorrhea; refer the athlete to a physician and have him refrain from all sexual contact

5.   During the rehabilitation of a knee injury, the athletic trainer decides the use of neuromuscular stimulation is indicated. As the athletic trainer is applying the electrodes to the athlete's thigh, the athlete says he has never had electric stimulation and is scared of electricity. Which of the following would be an appropriate response by the athletic trainer?
      A. Tell him he is being childish
      B. Demonstrate how it works on his coach
      C. Teach him about the general principles of electric stimulation
      D. Tell a joke about electricity to relax him

6.   A cross-country runner comes to you because he would like to begin a strength-training program for general body development. He informs you that he "has never really lifted weights before." How would you instruct him regarding his breathing pattern during a lift?
      A. Have the athlete inhale deeply at the beginning of the lift and then forcefully exhale at the end of the lift
      B. Have the athlete hold his breath during the lift
      C. Have the athlete inhale during the lift and hold his breath at the end of the lift
      D. Have the athlete breathe in, blow out, and breathe in again at the end of the lift

7.   When teaching an athlete how to properly use crutches, the athletic trainer should:
      A. Make sure the athlete's weight is fully supported on his or her hands and armpits
      B. Caution the athlete not to lean on the crutches so that his or her weight is on the crutch's axillary pads.
      C. Teach him or her how to use a cane first
      D. Teach the athlete a four-point gait

8.   A wrestler comes to the training room inquiring about a "drug that will make him lose weight quickly." He mentions a diuretic. Which of the following drugs has been banned by the International Olympic Committee (IOC) and causes diuresis?
      A. Furosemide
      B. Salbutamaol
      C. Caffeine (<12 mcg/mL)
      D. Salicylates

9. A baseball player complains of recurrent ingrown toenails. What might the athletic trainer suggest to prevent this problem?
    A. Have the athlete put a small amount of cotton under his nails
    B. Have the athlete wear shoes with a large toe-box
    C. Have the athlete trim his toenails in a rounded shape parallel to the border of the cuticle
    D. Have the athlete trim his toenails weekly and cut them straight across

10. When advising an athlete about the proper construction of a running shoe, which of the following criteria will help prevent foot and ankle injuries?
    I.   The midsole should be somewhat soft, but should not easily flatten out with pressure
    II. The shoe should have good forefoot flexibility
    III. The heel counter should be shallow and firm
    IV. The heel counter should be strong and fit well around the foot
    V.   The upper should be constructed of quality leather or rubber

    A. I, II, IV
    B. I, III, IV, V
    C. II, III, IV
    D. II, IV, V

11. You suspect one of your soccer players is experiencing "training staleness." Which of the following should you assess when developing a counseling approach with the athlete?
    A. The level of the athlete's ability to play the sport
    B. The relationship between the athlete and his family
    C. The athlete's training schedule and diet
    D. The athlete's competition schedule

12. When rehabilitating an athlete following a ligamentous wrist injury, once the ligament has healed enough where active motion can be initiated, it is important to educate the athlete to exercise only:
    A. Isometrically
    B. In water
    C. In a pain-free range
    D. First thing in the morning

13. To prevent the feeling of sedation during the day while taking medications for allergic rhinitis, the athletic trainer should suggest the athlete **not** take which of the following medications until he or she is ready to go to bed?
    A. Expectorants
    B. Antihistamines
    C. Decongestants
    D. NSAIDs

14. A varied diet that reflects a balance of the four food groups is important for an athlete to follow because:
    A. The athlete will maintain a healthy appetite
    B. Vitamin toxicity will be avoided
    C. Strict vegetarians tend to become anemic
    D. All of the above

15. To prevent the possibility of an acute compartment syndrome, the athletic trainer should advise his or her field hockey players to wear which of the following pieces of equipment?
    A. Shin guards
    B. Mouthguards
    C. Helmets
    D. Gloves

16. The dangers of possible hypothermia during exercise in very cold weather are significantly pronounced by_____ and _____.
    A. Light clothing, low chill factor
    B. Wind, wet weather
    C. Layered clothing, dry weather
    D. Wind, dry weather

17. One of your athletes has been diagnosed with Larsen-Johannson disease. Which of the following is **not** appropriate when advising the athlete in regard to minimizing his symptoms?
    A. To increase the strength of the VMO with isotonic quadriceps strengthening exercises
    B. Use ice packs frequently to minimize pain and swelling
    C. Avoid stressful activities such as running for approximately 6 months
    D. Avoid deep squatting

18. When counseling an athlete about the proper way to self-administer a medication, it is important that the athletic trainer make the athlete aware of what two factors?
    A. Any side effects and, in detail, how the drug works on the body
    B. If the drug may be addictive and how long the effects will last
    C. If the drug may cause depression and, in detail, how the drug works on the body
    D. When to take the medication and what foods/drugs not to mix with it

19. A female athlete should choose a sports bra that is supportive enough to prevent stretching of which structure?
    A. The skin
    B. The pectoralis major
    C. Cooper's ligament
    D. The nipples

20. An athlete experiences a catastrophic injury in which she is permanently unable to return to playing the only sport with which she is familiar. What would the appropriate response be by the athletic trainer when discussing the injury with the athlete?
    A. Tell her it is not appropriate to deny her condition and that it is best to accept her limitations
    B. Tell her it is OK for her to feel a variety of emotions and to openly express her needs and concerns
    C. Tell her to speak to her coach about her future in athletics
    D. Tell her to seek psychological counseling until she is no longer angry about her injury

21. When instructing an athlete in the proper technique of applying an elastic wrap to control pain and edema of an extremity, the athletic trainer should instruct the athlete to remove the wrap if all **except** the following occurs at the distal end of the extremity:
    A. Numbness
    B. Coolness
    C. Pink hue to the skin
    D. Cynanosis

22. An acronym used for the immediate care of an acute musculoskeletal injury is which of the following?
    A. ICER
    B. NSAID
    C. REST
    D. STAT

23. When advising an athlete about his year-long strength-training program, the athletic trainer should have the athlete limit his heavy lifting workouts to which periods?
    A. In-season and postseason
    B. Preseason and in-season
    C. Postseason and off-season
    D. Off-season and preseason

24. A swimmer reports to the athletic training room complaining of symptoms related to Scheurmann's disease. Which type of exercises is beneficial in trying to diminish the symptoms during the early stages of the disease?
    A. Cervical range of motion exercises
    B. Extension and postural exercises
    C. Williams' flexion exercises
    D. Houghston exercises

25. When rehabilitating an athlete following a lumbar strain, the athletic trainer should emphasize the significance of having the athlete improve the flexibility of all of the following structures **except**:
    A. The abdominals
    B. The iliopsoas
    C. The paraspinals
    D. The hamstrings

26. A drug that is used to increase the effect of another, such as aspirin when used in combination with codiene, is known as what kind of drug?
    A. Synergistic
    B. Cumulative
    C. Paradoxical
    D. Potentiating

27. When counseling an athlete about the adverse effects of anabolic steroids on females, all of the following effects should be included **except**:
    A. Severe acne
    B. Increased libido
    C. Increased body fat
    D. Development of a deep voice

28. You find out that a certified athletic trainer in your conference is selling an herbal substance to his athletes on a regular basis for personal profit. Which of the following codes is this individual violating?
    A. APTA Code of Honor
    B. NATA Code of Ethics
    C. NCAA Code of Honor
    D. ACSM Code of Medicine

29. What should the athletic trainer advise his or her athletes to do to minimize the negative effects of jet lag?
    A. Drink an adequate amount of fluids, especially water, to avoid dehydration
    B. Keep watches set to their "home" time zone
    C. Get up and go to bed 2 to 3 hours earlier for each time zone crossed
    D. Wear warm clothing to avoid getting cold while on the plane

30. Which of the following is **not** the proper action for an athlete to take if lightning is observed during a game?
    A. Avoid standing near metal bleachers on the field
    B. Stand near a telephone pole
    C. Assume a crouched position in a ditch
    D. Take cover in an automobile if the athlete cannot get indoors

31. You are aware of the general use of smokeless tobacco among your high school baseball players. You decide to develop a seminar for the coaches and players to discourage its use. Which of the following are effects of the chronic use of chewing tobacco?
    I.   Leukoplakia   IV. Bad breath
    II. Mouth and throat cancer V.   Mood swings
    III. Increased aggression   VI. Gynecomastia

    A. I, II, IV
    B. III, V, VI
    C. I, II, III
    D. II, III, IV

32. When explaining to a parent the difference between an athletic trainer and a physical therapist, the experitse of a physical therapist might best be decribed by which of the following?
    A. Expertise in the rehabilitation of the handicapped individual
    B. Those health care professionals trained in the rehabilitation of orthopedic injuries
    C. Those individuals trained in the rehabilitation of a diverse population
    D. Expertise in the rehabilitaion of athletic, geriatric, and neurologically impaired populations

33. Over the past 6 months, you notice one of the athletic trainers on your staff exhibiting some behaviors that are out of character for that individual. You recognize these behaviors as signs of "burnout." Which of the following are signs of job burnout?
    I. Insomnia
    II. Angry behavior
    III. Manic behavior
    IV. Self-preoccupation
    V. Attentiveness
    VI. Daily feelings of exhaustion

    A. I, II, IV, VI
    B. I, III, IV, V
    C. II, III, V, VI
    D. II, III, IV, VI

34. Which of the following is not among the best means by which an athletic trainer may educate the general public and other health care workers regarding the profession of athletic training?
    A. Organizing professional seminars and conferences
    B. Providing high quality care to the physically active individual
    C. Publishing articles in professional journals and participating in research
    D. Developing television advertisements

35. One of your basketball players comes into the athletic training room insisting that his ankles need to be taped even though he has no known injury. The athlete should be advised of which of the following?
    A. To let the trainer know if he starts developing any knee problems
    B. An elastic or neoprene ankle brace is more effective than taping in preventing an injury
    C. For the ankle taping to be effective, the athlete should rely on ankle-strengthening exercises rather than prophylactic taping if there is no injury present
    D. Advise the athlete to contact his family physician to evaluate his ankles

36. When taking a history from an athlete after an injury has occurred or when a problem arises, the most important thing an athletic trainer should do is:
    A. Be an active listener
    B. Make sure the athlete "gets to the point"
    C. Find out when the injury occurred
    D. Be sure to ask plenty of leading questions

37. One of your cross-country runners has an ongoing problem with tinea pedis. Which of the following actions should you take to assist this athlete in minimizing the problem?
    A. Use talcum powder daily and to keep his feet dry after showering
    B. Use Kwell shampoo twice a day or as directed by a physician
    C. Remove the infected toenail to prevent the infection from spreading
    D. Make sure the athlete uses sunblock with an SPF of 15 or higher

38. An athlete comes to the training room with what appears to be a tick embedded in his lower leg. The athletic trainer should instruct the athlete not to do which of the following?
    A. Keep the area clean and free of other debris
    B. Pull the tick off with tweezers
    C. Cover the tick with mineral oil
    D. Put fingernail polish onto its body

39. It is well-known that many athletes will utilize nutritional supplements in an effort to enhance performance. An athlete asks you to explain the action of an antioxidant. Which of the following best describes the role of an antioxidant?
    A. A nutrient that protects the cell from the detrimental effects of substances which may cause health problems, such as premature aging
    B. A mineral that is known to protect the body from cancer
    C. A vitamin that is known to protect the body from heart disease
    D. A substance that is found in vegetables and dairy products which prevents certain types of cancer and osteoporosis

40. One of your basketball players often complains about localized, lumbar "backaches." After performing your evaluation on this athlete, it appears his primary problem is postural. All of the following are actions that the athlete can take to prevent low back pain **except**:
    A. When standing for long periods of time, rest one foot on a stool if it is available
    B. Avoid sleeping in sidelying with the knees slightly bent
    C. Carry objects at waist level when possible
    D. Sit on chairs with a firm seat and straight back

41. In order to prevent medial epicondylitis, all of the following actions should be avoided via technique modification **except**:
    A. Too much wrist flexion at follow-through during a golf swing
    B. Excessive elbow valgus when throwing a javelin
    C. Hyperextension of the wrist when performing a backhand shot in tennis
    D. Excessive wrist flexion during a racquetball forehand shot

42. When assisting the general public in understanding the term "sports medicine," the definition should include which of the following descriptors?
    A. Strength training
    B. Physician
    C. Multidisciplinary
    D. Fitness

43. Which of the following individuals should the athletic trainer advise and consult with when developing a reconditioning program for an athlete following a musculoskeletal injury while playing football?
    A. The team strength and conditioning coach
    B. The school nurse
    C. The head football coach
    D. The athlete's parents if he is a minor

44. _____ and _____ are important qualities that an athletic trainer must possess when counseling an athlete during a time of distress.
    A. Empathy, humor
    B. Sympathy, pity
    C. Confidence, logic
    D. Objectivity, decisiveness

45. Which of the following qualities is necessary to be an effective educator in a student athletic training program?
    A. Competence in classroom teaching methods
    B. Competence in speech writing and communication skills
    C. A background in sociology
    D. Competence in computer language and audiovisual technology

Core Subject Areas

Athletic Training Evaluation

1. A _____ is a device used to measure joint range of motion.
   A. Goniometer
   B. Dynamometer
   C. Caliper
   D. Flexometer

2. Tenderness and pain with induration and swelling of the pretibial musculature following overexertion is indicative of which syndrome?
   A. Chondromalacia
   B. Pes anserine bursitis
   C. Shin splints
   D. Stress fracture

3. Speed's test is an evaluative test for which of the following problems:
   A. Thoracic outlet syndrome
   B. Supraspinatus tendinitis
   C. Bicipital tendinitis
   D. Ruptured biceps tendon

4. Who is the only person who can legally diagnose a medical problem?
   A. The school nurse
   B. A physician
   C. The athletic trainer
   D. An EMT or paramedic

5. If the calcaneofibular ligament of the ankle is torn, which of the following tests would be positive?
   A. Talar tilt test
   B. Anterior drawer sign
   C. Distraction test
   D. Clunk test

6. When taking a history during a physical examination of an athlete, all of the following information is pertinent **except**:
    A. The mechanism of the injury
    B. If a "pop" or "snap" was heard or felt
    C. If the athlete is on medication
    D. Whether or not the athlete has medical insurance

7. What problem might the athletic trainer see if the L4 nerve root was compressed?
    A. Hip flexor weakness
    B. Plantar flexion weakness
    C. Knee extension weakness
    D. Dorsiflexion weakness

8. With the athlete sitting and the scapula stabilized, the shoulder is maximally flexed; the athlete complains of pain and appears apprehensive. This is a positive _____ test.
    A. Yergason's
    B. Speed's
    C. Neer
    D. Compression

9. If a palpable "clunk" or shift at approximately 20° to 30° of knee flexion is found during a pivot-shift test, what may this be indicative of?
    A. Anterolateral rotary instability of the knee
    B. Anteromedial rotary instability of the knee
    C. Posterolateral rotary instability of the knee
    D. Posteromedial rotary instability of the knee

10. "Spearing" in football is a dangerous technique. Football coaches have discontinued this practice when teaching tackling techniques because it may cause severe head and neck injuries. What is the resulting force on the cervical spine when a football player spears an opponent?
    A. Sudden neck extension
    B. Sudden neck hyperflexion with rotation
    C. Sudden neck lateral flexion
    D. Sudden neck rotation

11. What is the most common mechanism of injury for an anterior shoulder dislocation?
    A. Adduction and external rotation
    B. Abduction and internal rotation
    C. Adduction and internal rotation
    D. Abduction and external rotation

12. Which of the following conditions often contributes to shoulder impingement?
    A. Acute bicipital tendinitis
    B. Suprascapular nerve entrapment
    C. Adhesive capsulitis
    D. Glenohumeral instability

13. An athlete has just been diagnosed with plantar fasciitis. All of the following would be appropriate measures to provide support/relief to the affected area **except**:
    A. An orthotic for arch support
    B. Lodi taping
    C. Metatarsal pad
    D. A heel cup

14. An athlete has been diagnosed with bulimia and has a known history of laxative abuse. Complications of chronic laxative use include which of the following problems?
    A. Electrolyte imbalance and dehydration
    B. Hyperactivity
    C. Hematemesis
    D. Chronic nasal congestion

15. An athlete comes to the athletic training room after being kicked in the lower leg by an opponent during a football game. He is complaining of decreased sensation in the L4 dermatome. What is this change in sensation called?
    A. Paresthesia
    B. Hypoesthesia
    C. Hyperesthesia
    D. Referred pain

16. _____ and _____ are two signs of diabetic coma.
    A. Drowsiness, acetone-smelling breath
    B. Seizures, pale and clammy skin
    C. Seizures, a bounding pulse
    D. Flushed skin, giddiness

17. Which of the following tests is used to detect a possible meniscal tear in the knee?
    A. Faber's test
    B. Allen test
    C. McMurray's test
    D. Lachman's test

18. An athlete reports to the athletic trainer with the presence of lesions on his upper lip and mouth area that look like blisters with a crusted yellow appearance and a red, weeping base. What is the probable cause of these lesions?
    A. Impetigo
    B. HIV
    C. Shingles
    D. A fungus infection

19. An athlete is brought to the athletic training room after sustaining a hard kick to the abdominal area. Which of the following symptoms is **not** a sign of a significant abdominal injury?
    A. Slow, deep respirations
    B. Increased heart rate, decreased blood pressure
    C. Ashen colored skin
    D. Rapid, shallow respirations

20. A football quarterback is sacked during a game. He comes off the field holding his throwing arm and complains of chest and anterior shoulder pain. After evaluating the athlete, the athletic trainer suspects a torn pectoralis major muscle. Which of the following physical findings will be seen if the athletic trainer is correct?
    A. Ecchymosis around the xiphoid process
    B. Palpable defect in the posterior axilla
    C. Weakness in abduction and external rotation
    D. Weakness in adduction, flexion, and internal rotation of the affected arm

21. While training in a high-altitude climate (eg, 9000 to 10,000 ft), a rock climber experiences acute dyspnea, cough, headache, and weakness. What is the probable cause of these symptoms?
    A. Asthma
    B. Pleurisy
    C. Bronchitis
    D. Pulmonary edema

22. A second-degree medial collateral ligament sprain is characterized by all of the following **except**:
    A. Pain along the medial joint line
    B. No gross knee instability, but mild ligamentous laxity is noted in full knee extension during valgus stress testing
    C. Difficulty in actively flexing and extending the knee
    D. Immediate, severe pain following the feeling of a "pop" in the knee. The pain quickly subsides and the athlete is left feeling a dull ache in the knee joint.

23. What is the usual mechanism of injury for a Colles' fracture?
    A. A fall on a closed fist
    B. A fall on a bent elbow
    C. A fall on an outstretched arm and hand
    D. A twisting movement of the knee when the lower leg is planted

24. What is the Allen test used for?
    A. To test the integrity of the vertebral arteries
    B. To test the integrity of the radial and ulnar arteries of the hand
    C. To test for carpal tunnel syndrome
    D. To test for thoracic outlet syndrome

25. Which of the carpal bones is most commonly dislocated?
    A. Scaphoid
    B. Lunate
    C. Cuboid
    D. Hamate

26. What type of force typically causes injury to the medial collateral ligament, medial meniscus, and anterior cruciate ligament of the knee?
    A. A valgus force with the tibia in external rotation
    B. A varus force with the knee in full extension
    C. A valgus force with the femur in external rotation
    D. A valgus force with the knee in recurvatum

27. An athlete sustains a neck injury during an ice hockey game and is complaining of numbness and tingling along with the ulnar border of his forearm and fourth and fifth fingers. Which of the following roentgenograms would be most appropriate in detecting nerve root compression?
    A. Electromyography or nerve root conduction velocity test
    B. CT scan or MRI
    C. Myelography
    D. Sonography

28. What of the following is an example of a "papule"?
    A. A freckle
    B. A wart
    C. A hive
    D. A friction blister

29. When testing for paresthesia of the C5 nerve root, where should the athletic trainer perform pinprick testing?
    A. Base of the neck
    B. At the nipple line
    C. The medial aspect of the arm
    D. The lateral aspect of the upper arm over the middle deltoid

30. What is the proper position to manually muscle test the anterior deltoid?
    A. Shoulder in full internal rotation with the palm facing the floor, the force directed downward
    B. Shoulder at 90° of abduction, full external rotation and supination with the force directed downward
    C. Resistance to the first 30° of abduction
    D. Arm at 90° of flexion, palm facing downward, and the force is in the downward direction

31. What is one of the most common symptoms of a lumbar discogenic injury?
    A. Dull, localized backache
    B. Localized swelling with muscle guarding
    C. Inability to backward bend
    D. Sharp, radiating pain down the back of the leg

32. When an athlete reports to the athletic trainer complaining of lateral hip pain, all of the following conditions might be the source of pain **except:**
    A. Trochanteric bursitis
    B. Strain of the gluteus medius
    C. Lumbar discogenic disease
    D. Avulsion of the ischial tuberosity

33. All of the following injuries might be associated with a "popping" sensation of the knee joint **except:**
    A. Anterior cruciate ligament injury
    B. Torn meniscus
    C. Subluxed patella
    D. Iliotibial band friction syndrome

34. The contact phase of the running gait is divided into which components?
    A. Forward swing and foot strike
    B. Foot strike, midsupport, and take-off
    C. Follow-through, forward swing, and foot descent
    D. Midsupport, take-off, and foot descent

35. Foot pronation results in _____ of the tibia during midsupport in the running gait.
    A. External rotation
    B. Internal rotation
    C. Abduction
    D. Adduction

36. A wrestler comes into the training room after sustaining a major elbow injury. There is intense pain, and the area is grossly swollen. The athlete is unable to straighten his elbow and the forearm appears shortened. The athletic trainer suspects an acute dislocation. Which two areas would the athletic trainer check for possible vascular impairment?
    A. Ulnar and radial pulses
    B. Radial pulse and color of the nailbeds after compression
    C. Brachial and radial pulses
    D. Arterial and venous circulation

37. An athlete sustains a blow to the head with a temporary loss of consciousness. He appears to have a lucid period where he seems to be normal for a period of a couple of hours and then becomes significantly lethargic. What type of medical emergency would the athletic trainer suspect?
    A. Ruptured intervertebral disc at level C3-4
    B. Extradural hemorrhage
    C. Basilar fracture
    D. Subdural hemorrhage

38. Concussions are usually graded on the _____ and _____ of neurologic impairment.
    A. Frequency, severity
    B. Frequency, duration
    C. Length, severity
    D. Duration, frequency

39. A tennis player comes to the athletic trainer complaining of medial thigh pain. He is limping and has pain with resisted hip adduction and hip flexion. There is diffuse tenderness and ecchymosis along the proximal aspect of the medial thigh. What is the probable cause of the pain?
    A. Hip flexor rupture
    B. Groin strain
    C. Medial hamstring strain
    D. Popliteus strain

40. A lacrosse player comes limping into the training room with assistance from a coach. He is holding his leg in slight hip and knee flexion. There is a large bulge in the proximal thigh. During the exam, the athletic trainer requests the athlete to extend his knee as he sits on the edge of a taping table. He is able to partially straighten his leg, although there is pain down the anterior thigh area with the attempt to move it. What does the athletic trainer suspect is wrong?
    A. Biceps femoris rupture
    B. Femoral nerve injury
    C. Ruptured rectus femoris muscle
    D. Obturator nerve injury

41. A basketball player reports to the training room complaining of a "burning" pain along the lateral aspect of his right knee during and after running. No edema or ecchymosis is found during the exam, but he is tender to palpation of the affected area. Which of the following special tests might be positive?
    A. Lachman's test
    B. Patellar apprehension test
    C. Ober test
    D. Sag sign

42. An athlete presents with loss of strength at the L3 and L4 nerve root levels. What muscle should the athletic trainer test to confirm an injury at this level?
    A. Quadriceps
    B. Flexor hallucis longus
    C. Gluteus maximus
    D. Adductor magnus

43. The athletic trainer asks an athlete to shrug his shoulders after a neck and shoulder injury. He has difficulty performing this movement even though it is not painful. What nerve is injured?
    A. Spinal accessory
    B. Dorsal scapular
    C. Long thoracic
    D. Suprascapular

44. How is the strength of the pes anserinus musculature manually muscle tested?
    A. Resistance to knee flexion and internal rotation of the lower leg
    B. Resistance to knee extension and hip adduction
    C. Resistance to knee flexion and external rotation of the lower leg
    D. Resistance to knee extension and internal rotation of the lower leg

45. During a track meet, you notice one of your runners appears somewhat disoriented. During your assessment of this athlete you find he is complaining of being light-headed, his skin is cool and clammy, he is sweating profusely, and his radial pulse is rapid. You take a rectal temperature and find it is mildly elevated (102° F). You suspect the athlete is suffering from which of the following problems?
    A. Heat cramps
    B. Prickly heat
    C. Heat stroke
    D. Heat exhaustion

46. One of your female gymnasts has been complaining of feeling generally fatigued on a constant basis. After being examined by the team physician, he orders a CBC (complete blood count). This blood test assesses all of the following **except**:
    A. Red blood cell count
    B. White blood cell count
    C. Plasma volume
    D. Hemoglobin levels

47. While elevating an athlete's shoulder, you note that the athlete is unable to abduct through the full range of motion against gravity. When performing a manual muscle test, this finding would be assigned which of the following muscle grades?
    A. 2+/5
    B. 3/5
    C. -4/5
    D. -3/5

48. You evaluate a basketball player who has sustained a finger injury while attempting to catch a ball. During your examination, you observe that the athlete is unable to extend the distal phalanx and the tip of his finger is positioned in approximately 30° of flexion. You determine the athlete has a mallet finger. This injury is caused by which of the following?
    A. Tenosynovitis of the abductor pollicis longus
    B. A subungual hematoma
    C. A sprain of the extensor pollicis brevis
    D. An avulsion of the extensor tendon from its insertion

49. During your examination of a football player who has sustained a low back injury during a tackle, you find that he is reporting dulled sensation along the dorsum of his right foot, he has difficulty walking on his heels, and his patellar tendon reflex is diminished. You suspect which of the following nerve root(s) is affected?
    A. L3
    B. L4
    C. L5
    D. S1-S3

50. When evaluating the inert structures of a joint, passive range of motion is used to determine all of the following **except**:
    A. The athlete's willingness to move
    B. Limitations of joint motion
    C. Joint stability
    D. Muscle and soft tissue elasticity

Human Anatomy

1. Inflammation of the common flexor origin of the forearm musculature is known as:
    A. Golfer's elbow
    B. Cycler's wrist
    C. Tennis elbow
    D. Pronation overuse syndrome

2. The olecranon process is located:
    A. On the ulna
    B. On the tibia
    C. On the vertebrae
    D. On the sternum

3. Which muscle does **not** assist in plantar flexion of the ankle?
    A. Peroneus tertius
    B. Posterior tibialis
    C. Plantaris
    D. Soleus

4. Which muscle does the axillary nerve innervate?
    A. Deltoid
    B. Latissimus dorsi
    C. Pectoralis minor
    D. Trapezius

5. The collateral ligaments of the knee are taut in:
    A. Flexion
    B. Extension
    C. Flexion and extension
    D. Genu varus

6. Which cranial nerve is injured if the athlete complains of a decrease in the sense of smell after a high velocity head injury?
    A. I
    B. IV
    C. III
    D. V

7. The rotator cuff consists of all the following muscles **except** the:
    A. Supraspinatus
    B. Infraspinatus
    C. Teres major
    D. Subscapularis

8. The rectus femoris muscle performs what two actions?
    A. Hip flexion and knee extension
    B. Hip extension and knee flexion
    C. Hip flexion and hip internal rotation
    D. Knee extension and hip internal rotation

9. The pes anserinus is made up of the tendons of what three muscles?
    A. Biceps femoris, gracilis, semitendinosis
    B. Iliotibial band, sartorious, semimembranous
    C. Sartorius, gracilis, semimembranous
    D. Sartorius, gracilis, semitendinosis

10. The subscapularis muscle originates on the _____ and inserts _____?
    A. Subscapular fossa, the lesser tubercle of the humerus
    B. Supraspinous fossa, the greater tubercle of the humerus
    C. Distal two thirds of the humerus, the coronoid process of the ulna
    D. Scapula, the middle third of the humerus

11. The gluteus maximus is responsible for the following motion(s):
    A. Flexion and internal rotation of the thigh
    B. Extension of the hip
    C External rotation of the hip
    D. External rotation and extension of the hip

12. What is the nerve root that affects elbow extension?
    A. C4
    B. C7
    C. C5
    D. C6

13. Holding a vibrating tuning fork next to the athlete's ear to determine air conduction of sound is a test for the _____ cranial nerve?
    A. VIII
    B. VI
    C. V
    D. X

14. To test the hypoglossal nerve, the athletic trainer should request the athlete to perform what action?
    A. Shrug his or her shoulders
    B. Stick his or her tongue out
    C. Open his or her mouth wide
    D. Smile

15. "Handlebar palsy," which occurs in cyclists, presents with motor weakness of what nerve(s)?
    A. Ulnar
    B. Median
    C. Musculocutaneous
    D. Ulnar and median

16. Where is the scaphoid bone of the wrist palpated?
    A. Proximal to the radial head
    B. Lateral to the cuboid bone
    C. Just distal to the styloid process of the radius
    D. Just distal to the styloid process of the ulna

17. All of the following muscles are innervated by the ulnar nerve **except:**
    A. Flexor carpi ulnaris
    B. Adductor pollicis
    C. All the hypothenar muscles
    D. Extensor carpi ulnaris

18. What type of joint is the hip joint?
    A. Fibrous
    B. Amphiarthrotic
    C. Synarthrotic
    D. Diarthrotic

19. Flexion and extension of the knee joint occurs in the _____ plane around a _____ axis.
    A. Sagittal, transverse
    B. Sagittal, coronal
    C. Frontal, anterior-posterior
    D. Transverse, longitudinal

20. Which of the following describes an impacted fracture?
    A. A fracture that telescopes one part of the bone on the other
    B. The bone splits along its length
    C. The fracture is at a right angle to the shaft
    D. A fracture consisting of three or more fragments at the fracture site

21. Which of the following joints is classified as a uniaxial diarthrodial joint?
    A. The interphalangeal joints of the fingers
    B. Hip joint
    C. Carpometacarpal joint of the thumb
    D. Scapulothoracic joint

22. Which of the following muscles does **not** flex the hip?
    A. Biceps femoris
    B. Pectineus
    C. Iliopsoas
    D. Rectus femoris

23. Which of the following movements are the greatest in the thoracic region?
    A. Lateral flexion of the spine
    B. Flexion and extension of the spine
    C. Rotation and extension of the spine
    D. Flexion of the spine

24. Which structures are located in the lateral compartment of the lower leg?
    A. Extensor digitorum longus, peroneus longus, and peroneus brevis muscles
    B. Peroneus longus and brevis muscles, the superficial branch of the peroneal nerve, and the peroneal artery
    C. Posterior tibialis muscle, posterior tibial artery, and the deep peroneal nerve
    D. Extensor digitorum longus, peroneal brevis, and peroneal tertius muscles

25. Where would a Baker's cyst be located?
    A. In the popliteal fossa
    B. In the groin area
    C. On the breast
    D. On the lip

26. Which of the joints below comprise the shoulder girdle?
    I. Sternoclavicular   IV. Scapulothoracic
    II. Acromioclavicular   V. Costoclavicular
    III. Glenohumeral   VI. Scapulohumeral

    A. I, II, VI
    B. I, II, III, IV
    C. III, IV, V, VI
    D. III, V, VI

27. The coracoclavicular ligaments consist of the _____ and _____ ligaments.
    A. Trapezoid, conoid
    B. Coracoacromial, conoid
    C. Acromioclavicular, trapezoid
    D. Costoclavicular, conoid

28. Which of the following joints is a "mortise" joint?
    A. First metatarsophalangeal joint
    B. Elbow
    C. Ankle
    D. Knee

29. What two structures pass through the tunnel of Guyon?
    A. The ulnar nerve and ulnar artery
    B. The radial and ulnar nerves
    C. The radial nerve and radial artery
    D. The ulnar nerve and radial artery

30. Which muscle is usually affected with tennis elbow?
    A. Extensor carpi radialis brevis
    B. Flexor carpi radialis
    C. Extensor carpi ulnaris
    D. Extensor pollicis brevis

31. All of the following muscles are intrinsic muscles of the hand **except**:
    A. The lumbricals
    B. The muscles of the thenar eminence
    C. The interossei
    D. The multifidi muscles

32. What are the primary actions of the psoas major?
    A. Abduction of the hip
    B. Extension and internal rotation of the hip
    C. Hip flexion and internal rotation
    D. Trunk flexion

33. Where is the origin of the vastus lateralis located?
    A. Gerdy's tubercle
    B. The anterior inferior iliac spine
    C. The greater trochanter of the femur
    D. The lateral aspect of the femur

34. Which of the following muscle tendons form the boundaries of the anatomical snuff-box?
    I.   Extensor hallucis longus   IV. Abductor pollicis longus
    II. Extensor pollicis brevis   V.   Extensor pollicis longus
    III. Flexor pollicis longus

    A. I, III, V
    B. I, II, IV
    C. III, IV, V
    D. II, IV, V

35. The structure that carries deoxygenated blood from the head and upper body to the heart is the:
    A. Descending aorta
    B. Superior vena cava
    C. Ascending aorta
    D. Jugular vein

36. At which of the following structures does gas exchange occur in the lungs?
    A. Terminal bronchiole
    B. The parietal pleura
    C. The alveoli
    D. The pulmonary veins

37. All of the following structures pass through the popliteal fossa **except**:
    A. Tibial nerve
    B. Popliteal artery
    C. Popliteal vein
    D. Peroneal artery

38. Where is the odontoid process located?
    A. Base of the sacrum
    B. Proximal end of the ulna
    C. Off the second cervical vertebrae
    D. Base of the skull

39. Which of the following bones is **not** a carpal bone of the wrist?
    A. Lunate
    B. Cuneiform
    C. Hamate
    D. Pisiform

40. The plantar fascia or plantar aponeurosis is located where in the body?
    A. Base of the neck
    B. Lumbar region
    C. Lateral side of the thigh
    D. Sole of the foot

41. The sternocleidomastoid muscle originates on the _____ and inserts into the _____.
    A. Mastoid process, clavicle
    B. Clavicle and sternum, mastoid process
    C. Manubrium, occipital protuberance
    D. Manubrium, clavicle

42. Which of the following muscles is a strong extensor of the trunk?
    A. Gluteus maximus
    B. Erector spinae
    C Quadratus lumborum
    D. Iliacus

43. Which structures pass through the femoral triangle?
    A. Femoral artery, femoral vein, femoral nerve
    B. Femoral artery, femoral nerve, iliac vein
    C. Deep circumflex vein, femoral nerve
    D. Great saphenous vein, femoral vein, iliac vein

44. Which artery is closely involved with the brachial plexus and becomes the brachial artery at the lower border of the tendon of the teres major muscle?
    A. Subclavian artery
    B. Radial artery
    C. Axillary artery
    D. Subscapular artery

45. Which of the following muscles does **not** dorsiflex the ankle?
    A. Extensor digitorum longus
    B. Peroneus tertius
    C. Tibialis anterior
    D. Peroneus brevis

46. Which of the following is **not** a bone of the middle ear?
    A. Malleus
    B. Cochlea
    C. Stapes
    D. Incus

47. Where is the C3-4 dermatome located?
    A. The top of the head
    B. Over the posterior upper arm area
    C. Over the lateral upper arm area
    D. The superior aspect of the shoulders and posterior neck area

48. In what abdominal quadrant is the spleen located?
    A. Upper left
    B. Lower right
    C. Lower left
    D. Upper right

49. Your athlete comes to the training room after injuring his neck and left arm. You suspect involvement of the C5-6 nerve root. Which of the following actions would **not** be involved with an injury to a muscle with this innervation?
    A. Little finger abduction
    B. Elbow flexion
    C. Shoulder abduction
    D. Forearm supination

50. A soccer player has been kicked in the upper right quadrant of his abdomen. Which of the following internal organ(s) could have sustained a significant injury?
    A. Kidney
    B. Liver, gallbladder
    C. Spleen
    D. Appendix, sigmoid colon

Human Physiology

1. The bottom number of a blood pressure reading is the _____ pressure.
    A. Diastolic
    B. Systolic
    C. Ejection fraction
    D. Venous

2. The optimum time an ice pack should be applied to a body part is 10 minutes. This is to avoid the _____ response.
    A. Vasomotor
    B. Blocking
    C. Moro
    D. Hunting

3. Redness and swelling during the inflammation process is caused by all of the following **except**:
    A. Histamine
    B. Prostaglandins
    C. Serotonin
    D. Acetylcholine

4. What is the level of desirable total cholesterol?
    A. Less than or equal to 200 mg/100 mL
    B. Greater than 250 mg/100 mL
    C. 55 mg/100 mL
    D. Less than 100 mg/100 mL

5. The separation of electrically charged particles causing a transmembrane electrical potential difference is known as:
    A. Resting membrane potential
    B Membrane permeability threshold
    C. Electrogenic pump
    D. Depolarization threshold

6. When sodium ions move into a cell and the transmembrane potential is reduced (approaches zero), and when potassium ions rush out of the cell and the transmembrane potential is gradually reestablished, an action potential is created. The two phases described above are known as:
    A. Depolarization/repolarization
    B. Repolarization/depolarization
    C. Stimulation/propagation
    D. Propagation/repolarization

7. The primary component of striated skeletal muscle is the:
    A. Sarcomere
    B. Muscle fiber
    C. Myofibril
    D. Fascicle

8. What does a motor unit consist of?
    A. A cell body, axon, and dendrites
    B. The axon and single muscle fiber it innervates
    C. A motor neuron and the group of muscle fibers it innervates
    D. The motor neuron, muscle fiber, and muscle group

9. What type of muscle fiber is more prevalent in a sprinter s lower extremity?
    A. Fast twitch
    B. Type I
    C. Slow twitch
    D. Smooth

10. What mineral must be present in adequate amounts in the muscle fiber for a contraction to occur?
    A. Na+
    B. Ca++
    C. Cl-
    D. PO_4

11. In addition to the release of energy, the breakdown of ATP during a muscle contraction produces which of the following byproducts?
    A. $H_2O + CO_2$
    B. $Cr + PO_4$
    C. $ADP + PO_4$
    D. ADP + ATPASE

12. During aerobic metabolism, enzymes reduce large molecules of carbohydrates, fat, and protein into smaller particles so they can be oxidized in a chain of chemical reactions. These series of chemical reactions are collectively known as:
    A. The Krebs cycle
    B. Oxidative carboxylic acid cycle
    C. Thermocaloric cycle
    D. Phosphocreatine reaction

13. Deep pain may originate from three specific areas when a nerve is injured. These areas are known as sclerotomes, myotomes, and dermatomes. Sclerotomic pain is transported by what type of nerve fiber?
    A. Unmyelinated C fibers
    B. Unmyelinated D fibers
    C. Myelinated A-Delta fibers
    D. Myelinated C fibers

14. Muscular fiber arrangements may be known as _____ or _____.
    A. Fusiform, pennate
    B. Oblique, striated
    C. Striated, smooth
    D. Multinuclear, uninuclear

15. What is amenorrhea?
    A. Diminished flow during menses
    B. Absence of flow during menses
    C. Painful menses
    D. Late onset of menses

16. What should be avoided with an athlete who has frequent episodes of constipation?
    A. Laxatives or enemas
    B. High fiber diet
    C. Bland diet
    D. Calcium supplements

17. Hemophilia occurs when which of the following blood factors is missing?
    A. Granulocytes
    B. Hemoglobin
    C. Factor IV
    D. Factor VIII

18. In addition to the partial pressure of oxygen in the alveolar gas of the lungs, what other factors influence the rate of diffusion of oxygen into the bloodstream?
    A. The respiratory rate and pleural surface area
    B. The amount of CO_2 present in the alveoli and the pulmonary veins
    C. The respiratory rate and CO_2 partial pressure
    D. The thickness of the alveolar capillary membrane and the amount of surface area available for diffusion

19. An athlete's pulmonary function is tested via spirometry. Several measurements are taken during this test. The maximum amounts of air that can be expired after a maximum inspiration is known as:
    A. Maximum expiratory flow rate
    B. Forced expiratory volume
    C. Vital capacity
    D. Tidal volume

20. During what phase of the menstrual cycle does a graafian follicle mature?
    A. Follicular
    B. Ovulatory
    C. Luteal
    D. Menstrual

21. What are the two phases of menstruation?
    A. Anovulation, luteal
    B. Prolactin, menarche
    C. Follicular, luteal
    D. Menarche, follicular

22. Which of the following structures is **not** innervated?
    A. Periosteum of bone
    B. Peritoneum of the abdomen
    C. Epithelium of the skin
    D. Enamel of a tooth

23. A football player sustained a large laceration to his lower leg 4 weeks ago. Which type of repair has taken place by this time?
    A. Callus formation
    B. Primary healing
    C. Margination
    D. Secondary healing

24. Noxious stimuli that are created by musculoskeletal injury result in the release of endorphins and enkephalins during the mediation of pain. These opioids are produced by the stimulation of the _____ of the midbrain and _____ in the pons and medulla.
    A. Periaqueductal gray area, substantia gelatinosa
    B. Periaqueductal gray area, raphe nucleus
    C. Central cortex, substantia gelatinosa
    D. Raphe nucleus, red nucleus

25. A female field hockey player reports to the athletic trainer complaining that her knee still hurts from a grade II medial collateral ligament sprain she suffered almost 3 months ago. How long may it take for a ligament to completely heal after a significant injury?
    A. Between 4 and 6 months
    B. Up to 1 year
    C. Up to 4 months
    D. Between 1.5 and 2 years

26. You are aware of a diabetic athlete who has just self-administered his morning dose of insulin and has basketball practice within the following hour. Which of the following would be a prudent action to suggest to this athlete before he begins exercising?
    A. Hyperhydrate prior to practice
    B. Eat a candy bar before practice
    C. Suggest the athlete eat a slice of bread with peanut butter or cheese prior to practice
    D. Drink a soft drink before exercising

27. All of the following are physiological responses to cryotherapy **except**:
    A. Increased metabolism
    B. Decreased muscle spasm
    C. Analgesia
    D. Increased joint stiffness

28. An athlete falls on an outstretched hand and injures his wrist. After evaluating the injury, the athletic trainer suspects a scaphoid fracture. Because this area has a poor blood supply, which of the following conditions may occur if the injury is mistreated?
    A. DeQuervain's syndrome
    B. Aseptic necrosis
    C. Carpal tunnel syndrome
    D. Swan neck deformity

29. A soccer player gets kicked in the low back and is brought to the training room. During his examination, he goes to the bathroom and reports that there is blood in his urine. Which of the following terms describes this sign of an internal injury?
    A. Hyperpnea
    B. Hematoma
    C. Hematuria
    D. Hemarthrosis

30. Smooth muscle tissue is found in all the following structures **except**:
    A. Lungs
    B. Arterial walls
    C. Scalenes
    D. Intestines

31. While performing an isometric contraction, an athlete should be instructed to breathe normally to prevent the valsalva effect. Which of the following occurs when the athlete produces the valsalva effect?
    A. The athlete experiences dyspnea
    B. The athlete will hyperventilate
    C. The athlete becomes hypotensive
    D. There is a significant, rapid rise in blood pressure

32. During ballistic stretching, the golgi tendon organs are unable to produce a relaxing effect of the muscle because of the constant stimulation of which of the following structures?
    A. Muscle spindles
    B. Posterior horn of the spinal cord
    C. The antagonist muscle
    D. Cerebral cortex

33. The adrenal glands secrete which of the following substances?
    I.   Cortisol   IV. Aldosterine
    II. Epinephrine   V. Estrogen
    III. Serotonine   VI. Human growth hormone

    A. I, II, III, VI
    B. I, II, IV, V
    C. II, III, V, VI
    D. III, IV, V, VI

34. A male athlete gets kicked in the groin area and sustains an injury to the testicles. The major function of the testes is to produce _____ and _____.
    A. Semen, urine
    B. Spermatozoa, testosterone
    C. Testosterone, estrogen
    D. Semen, spermatozoa

Exercise Physiology

1. The training effect on the cardiac system can be defined as:
   A. CO = increased SV + decreased HR
   B. CO = SV / HR
   C. CO = decreased SV increased HR
   D. SV = CO x HR

2. When reading an exercise prescription, which of the following statements represents the frequency of exercise?
   A. Three sessions a week
   B. 45 minutes of continuous exercises
   C. Running or cycling
   D. 80% of VO_2 max

3. Total cholesterol is made up of three different lipoproteins. These include:
   A. Triglycerides, HDL, and LDL
   B. LDL, HDL, and VLDL
   C. LDL, VLDL, and triglycerides
   D. Alpha lipoprotein, LDL, and triglycerides

4. During vigorous activity, accessory muscles come into play to aid respiration. During inspiration, these muscles include the _____ and _____.
   A. Upper trapezius, levator scapulae
   B. Sternocleidomastoids, scalenes
   C. Intercostals, abdominals
   D. Intercostals, levator scapulae

5. In very cold environments, the athlete's body will attempt to produce heat through many different mechanisms. One of these methods is by hypothalamic stimulation of:
    A. Posterior hypothalamus
    B. Sweat glands
    C. Thyroid gland
    D. Adrenal glands

6. A basketball player comes limping off the court complaining of a hamstring spasm. Which of the following procedures would be the most effective in reducing the spasm?
    A. Massage the hamstring
    B. Moist heat pack followed by ultrasound
    C. Static stretch of the involved muscle
    D. Static stretch of the antagonistic muscle

7. An athlete who is hyperflexible (mobile beyond the joint's normal range) is subject to what types of injuries?
    A. Tendinitis, bursitis
    B. Fractures, ligament tears
    C. Sprains, strains
    D. Subluxations, dislocations

8. Interval training would be appropriate for all the following sports **except**:
    A. Football
    B. Soccer
    C. Archery
    D. Basketball

9. During what season would it be beneficial for an athlete to participate in a sport (other than his or her primary sport) to maintain an adequate level of fitness?
    A. Off-season
    B. Postseason
    C. In-season
    D. Preseason

10. When designing a training program for an athlete, which of the following principles must be adhered to in order to obtain optimal training effects?
    I.   Overload   IV. Consistency
    II. Specificity   V. Environmental factors
    III. Progression   VI. Psychological wellbeing

    A. I, III, IV, V
    B. II, IV, V, VI
    C. I, II, III, IV
    D. II, III, V, VI

11. All of the following effects are true regarding changes that take place as a result of resistive exercise **except:**
    A. Increased ligament and tendon strength
    B. Improved elasticity of skeletal muscle
    C. Increased mineral content of bone
    D. Improved maximal oxygen uptake

12. Under which of the following conditions is the tension created in a muscle the greatest during exercise?
    A. When the interaction between the cross-bridges of the actin and myosin myofilaments are at a maximum
    B. When the muscle position is at its shortest
    C. When a muscle is at its most lengthened point
    D. When the muscle insertion is at a 90° angle to the shaft of a bone

13. _____ and _____ determine the amount of blood that is pumped through the heart in a given period of time.
    A. Cardiac output, heart rate
    B. Respiratory rate, ventricular filling rate
    C. Stroke volume, cardiac output
    D. Heart rate, stroke volume

14. If a 20-year-old athlete is exercising at 80% of his maximal heart rate; his target heart rate could be calculated to equal:
    A. 150 BPM
    B. 160 BPM
    C. 170 BPM
    D. 200 BPM

15. In order to improve an athlete's flexibility, PNF techniques may be incorporated into a training program. Which of the following techniques involves an isotonic contraction during the "push" phase?
    A. Hold-relax
    B. Contract-relax
    C. Slow-reversal-hold-relax
    D. Fast-reversal-hold-relax

16. When bench-pressing a barbell, the triceps and pectoralis major musculature contract in what manner during the "lift" phase?
    A. Isokinetically
    B. Isometrically
    C. Eccentrically
    D. Concentrically

17. Which type of training program is most beneficial if the coach or athletic trainer is trying to improve muscular strength and flexibility?
    A. Plyometric training
    B. Anaerobic training
    C. Circuit training
    D. Power lifting

18. If an athlete is **not** well-hydrated and is in poor physical condition in the beginning of a sport season, and he is exercising in a very hot, humid environment, he may be susceptible to heat injuries. What is the area of the body that is responsible for thermoregulation?
    A. Barioceptors
    B. Thymus
    C. Hypothalamus
    D. Pituitary gland

19. Year-round sports conditioning is developed through the concept of periodization. Periodization is an approach that allows the athlete to train in stages so peak performance may be attained at the appropriate time and injuries are avoided. Which of the following describe the different phases in periodization?
    A. Fall season, winter season, spring season, off-season
    B. Postseason, off-season, preseason, in-season
    C. First, second, third, and forth quarters
    D. Preparation phase, active phase, maintenance phase

20. The purpose of a proper cool-down period after exercising is to _____ and _____.
    A. Decrease the heart rate, decrease cardiac output
    B. Increase ventilation, prevent dizziness
    C. Help the blood return to the heart to be reoxygenated, decrease muscular lactic acid build-up
    D. Improve flexibility, decrease body temperature

21. Which type of exercise utilizes a rapid stretch of the muscle eccentrically followed by a rapid concentric contraction and is used to develop explosive movements?
    A. Plyometric exercise
    B. Isokinetic exercise
    C. Isotonic exercise
    D. Internal exercise

22. Developing significant muscle bulk is dependent on the levels present in the body of which of the following hormones?
    A. Epinephrine
    B. Cortisol
    C. Testosterone
    D. Estrogen

23. To help prevent an athlete from developing hypothermia while playing in very cold weather, what should the athletic trainer advise the athlete to do?
    A. Wear a hooded sweatshirt
    B. Only stay out in the cold for brief periods of time
    C. Wear layers of clothing
    D. Wear lined pants

24. One of your lacrosse players has blonde hair, light green eyes, and a very fair complexion. You suggest she wear a sunscreen with which of the following levels of sun protection factor (SPF)?
    A. 4
    B. 6
    C. 10
    D. 30

25. An asthmatic athlete who lives and trains in an urban area is susceptible to the effects of air pollution. To avoid an asthma attack while training, the athletic trainer should recommend that the athlete train at which of the following times of day?
    A. Predawn hours
    B. Mid-day
    C. Late afternoon
    D. On weekends and the evening

26. You have an African-American athlete with known sickle-cell disease who is training in high altitudes for a long distance road race. What condition might this athlete be at risk for?
    A. Ruptured spleen
    B. Enlarged gallbladder
    C. Cystic fybrosis
    D. Tinea corporis

27. Unlimited access to fluids is critical during hot weather because the athlete will sweat more. Sweat is hypotonic, which means what imbalance is the athlete likely to experience?
    A. Water loss in excess of salt loss
    B. Salt loss in excess of water loss
    C. Water loss is equal to salt loss
    D. Sugar loss in excess of water loss

28. Delayed-onset muscle soreness (DOMS) can occur with high-intensity exercise. Which of the following types of exercise is most likely to cause DOMS?
    A. Endurance
    B. Isometric
    C. Plyometric
    D. PNF

29. If a joint capsule is stretched beyond its physiological limitations causing a reflexive muscle contraction, which of the following laws is being demonstrated?
    A. Ohm's law
    B. Hilton's law
    C. Wolff's law
    D. Newton's law

30. When performing a urinalysis with a dipstick (such as Clinix Stix or a similar product) for abnormal glucose and protein levels, which of the following are considered abnormal findings in the adolescent?
    A. +2
    B. +3
    C. +4
    D. All of the above

31. Men are generally much stronger than women because:
    A. Women have a lower strength : body weight ratio
    B. Men have a lower strength : body weight ratio
    C. Men have a greater strength : muscle mass ratio
    D. Women have a greater strength : fat percentage ratio

32. Which of the following physiological adaptations do **not** occur in skeletal muscle during endurance training?
    A. Increased aerobic enzyme activity
    B. Increased myoglobin levels
    C. Increased mitochondrial density
    D. Decreased mitochondrial density

33. During a 400-meter sprint, which of the following energy systems is predominant?
    A. Lactic acid system
    B. ATP-CP system
    C. Anaerobic glycolysis
    D. Aerobic metabolic system

34. What effect does aerobic exercise have on an athlete's diastolic blood pressure?
    A. Diastolic blood pressure will increase at the same pace as systolic
    B. Diastolic blood pressure will significantly decrease at higher work loads
    C. It will remain closely the same level as at rest
    D. Diastolic blood pressure will significantly increase with increasing workloads

35. Footstrike anemia can be controlled by having the athlete wear well-cushioned shoes, limiting running to very soft surfaces, and teaching the athlete to land lightly on his or her feet while exercising. This condition is also known as:
    A. Hemolysis
    B. Hyperkalemia
    C. Rubefacients
    D. Hemarthrosis

Biomechanics

1. A contraction that occurs as the muscle shortens is known as:
   A. Isotonic
   B. Eccentric
   C. Isometric
   D. Concentric

2. The foot becomes a "rigid lever" for push-off when it is in what position?
   A. Supination
   B. Pronation
   C. Dorsiflexion
   D. Adduction

3. How many degrees of freedom does the knee have?
   A. 1°
   B. 2°
   C. 3°
   D. 4°

4.   How many degrees of movement does the scapula contribute to shoulder abduction?
     A. 30°
     B. 60°
     C. 100°
     D. 180°

5.   During active knee extension against gravity, the quadriceps musculature assumes what role?
     A. Antagonist
     B. Agonist
     C. Synergist
     D. Stabilizer

6.   In the human body, the point of attachment of the muscle causing the motion is almost always closer to the joint axis than the resisting motion. What type of lever system most commonly exists in the body?
     A. First
     B. Second
     C. Third
     D. Fourth

7.   In what position will the movement arm of a force be the greatest?
     A. When the movement arm is at a 45° angle to the applied force
     B. When the force of gravity is 90° to the applied force
     C. When the lever being moved is parallel to the applied force
     D. When the angle of application of the force is at 90° to the lever being moved

8.   Of the following statements, which is true about anatomic pulleys?
     A. Anatomic pulleys change the direction of the muscle force, but not the magnitude of the force
     B. Anatomic pulleys always deflect the line of pull of a muscle away from the joint axis
     C. Anatomic pulleys change the direction and magnitude of the force
     D. Anatomic pulleys improve leverage, and therefore increase the magnitude of the force

9.   Muscular tension may be increased by increasing the _____ or _____.
     A. Frequency of motor units firing, the number of motor units that are stimulated
     B. External force, inert muscle force
     C. Contractile tension, viscoelastic tension
     D. Number of repetitions while weight lifting, the poundage of weight

10. What three motions comprise pronation of the foot?
     A. Inversion, abduction, dorsiflexion
     B. Inversion, adduction, plantar flexion
     C. Eversion, abduction, dorsiflexion
     D. Eversion, adduction, plantar flexion

11. What class lever does the gastrocnemius use during plantar flexion?
     A. First
     B. Second
     C. Third
     D. Fourth

12. Each lever has a _____, which is the perpendicular distance from the line of force to the axis, and a _____, which is the perpendicular distance from the resistance to the axis.
    A. Force arm, rotary arm
    B. Short arm, long arm
    C. Force arm, resistance arm
    D. Rotary arm, translatory arm

13. Running utilizes _____ motion of the entire body and _____ motion of the arms and legs.
    A. Decelerant, accelerant
    B. Vertical, horizontal
    C. Rotary, translatory
    D. Linear, angular

14. Momentum is created by the combination of _____ and _____.
    A. Speed, weight
    B. Mass, velocity
    C. Acceleration, weight
    D. Torque, friction

15. A sprinter who is in the "ready" position at the start of a race has a lot of potential energy. As he takes off when the gun is heard, his potential energy is converted into:
    A. Lactic acid
    B. Thermal energy
    C. Work energy
    D. Kinetic energy

16. Which of the following describes the plane and axis for cervical rotation?
    A. Horizontal, vertical
    B. Horizontal, sagittal
    C. Sagittal, anterior-posterior
    D. Frontal, vertical

17. When manually resisting the tibia during knee extension, all of the following statements regarding the torque produced are true **except**:
    A. The torque of an external force (ie, the hand against the anterior tibia) can be increased by increasing the magnitude of the applied force
    B. The torque of an external force can be increased by applying the force perpendicular to the tibial crest
    C. The torque of an external force can be increased by moving the force distally near the ankle
    D. The torque of an external force can be increased by applying the force parallel to the tibial shaft

18. An avulsion fracture of a bone is caused by which type of tissue stress?
    A. Compression
    B. Bending
    C. Shearing
    D. None of the above

19. A lever is considered in rotational equilibrium when any muscle acting on that lever is neither short-ening nor lengthening. This results in what kind of contraction?
     A. Isometric
     B. Isotonic
     C. Passive
     D. Concentric

20. What type of joint is the carpometacarpal joint of the thumb?
     A. Pivot joint
     B. Saddle joint
     C. Hinge joint
     D. Plane joint

21. What is the maximum degrees of freedom a joint can possess?
     A. 2°
     B. 3°
     C. 4°
     D. 6°

22. Which of the following joints is an example of a hinge joint?
     A. Acromioclavicular joint
     B. Atlantoaxial joint
     C. Elbow joint
     D. Shoulder joint

23. The frontal plane divides the body into _____ and _____ parts.
     A. Top, anterior
     B. Right, left
     C. Top, bottom
     D. Anterior, posterior

24. What is an example of an activity taking place with the upper extremity in a closed-chain position?
     A. Swinging a bat
     B. Performing a push-up
     C. Throwing a ball
     D. Running with closed fists

25. What occurs at the knee joint during the screw-home mechanism?
     A. The tibia externally rotates on the femur during knee extension
     B. The femur externally rotates on the tibia during knee flexion
     C. The femur internally rotates on the tibia during knee extension
     D. The tibia internally rotates on the femur during knee extension

26. What occurs at the articulating surfaces of a joint that is subjected to a compressive load?
     A. The joint surfaces are brought closer together
     B. The joint surfaces are forcefully separated
     C. There is a "twisting" movement at the joint surfaces
     D. There is a "bending" motion that occurs at the joint surfaces

27. Loading of a joint that is unstable due to a ligament rupture produces which of the following stresses on the joint cartilage?
    A. No change at all
    B. Abnormally low stress
    C. Tension forces
    D. None of the above

28. Shoulder abduction occurs in the _____ plane and moves around a _____ axis.
    A. Frontal, sagittal
    B. Horizontal, vertical
    C. Frontal, anterior-posterior
    D. Sagittal, medial-lateral

29. Hip internal/external rotation occurs in the _____ plane around a _____ axis.
    A. Sagittal, medial-lateral
    B. Horizontal, anterior-posterior
    C. Frontal, anterior-posterior
    D. Horizontal, vertical

30. While covering a football game, a player gets tackled and sustains a spiral fracture of the tibial shaft. Which of the following force(s) comes into play when a bone is fractured in this manner?
    A. Compression, tension
    B. Torsion
    C. Compression, shearing
    D. Impaction

31. Repeated rubbing over the epidermis may cause which of the following conditions?
    A. Avulsion
    B. Blisters
    C. Contusions
    D. Bursitis

Psychology

1. An athlete comes to the athletic trainer just prior to his first soccer game complaining of nausea and informs the trainer he is really nervous. Which of the following is an appropriate method to relax a nervous athlete?
    A. Yoga
    B. Progressive muscle relaxation
    C. Have the coach calm the athlete
    D. Resting in a warm sauna for 10 minutes

2. The coach confers with the athletic trainer concerning a difficult athlete on his team. During his description of the athlete's behavior, he complains of the athlete's lack of assertiveness, procrastination, constant criticism of others, and evasiveness. What type of behavior does this profile?
    A. Obsessive-compulsive
    B. Passive-aggressive
    C. Anxiety disorder
    D. Depression

3. Which of the behaviors below are seen with abuse of anabolic steroids?
    I.   Mania   IV. Psychosis
    II. Depression   V. Hyperactivity
    III. Anxiety   VI. Insomnia

    A. III, V, VI
    B. I, II
    C. V, VI
    D. I, II, III, VI

4. Which of the following is **not** a stage of the general adaptation syndrome (response phases of stress)?
    A. Exhaustion
    B. Anger
    C. Resistance
    D. Alarm

5. An athlete who is burned out may display which of the following symptoms?
    A. Negative self-concept
    B. Chronic fatigue
    C. Negative attitude toward his teammates
    D. All of the above

6. At the time of injury the athlete experiences a great deal of stress. The athlete responds to this stressor by passing through three psychophysiological phases. During which of the following phases are the adrenal glands most active?
    A. Exhaustive
    B. Resistance
    C. Anger
    D. Alarm

7. You notice one of your basketball players is showing signs of overtraining. Which of the following would **not** be an appropriate response to an overtrained athlete by the athletic trainer?
    A. Listening to the athlete's fears
    B. A tapered decrease in training over a period of 1 week
    C. An abrupt cessation of training
    D. Counseling the athlete in relaxation techniques

8. Which of the following must the athlete feel if he or she is to have a good rapport with the athletic trainer?
    A. Trust
    B. Empathy
    C. Pity
    D. Love

9. How might an athletic trainer assist the athlete in helping him- or herself heal after an injury?
    A. Provide the athlete access to painkillers
    B. Help the athlete "visualize" the healing process through imagery
    C. Give the athlete articles to read about his or her injury
    D. Make sure therapeutic modalities are applied in the correct sequence

10. After a wrestler is injured, you notice he has developed a very negative attitude and is generally depressed. Two methods of redirecting this athlete's negative and angry ideas are _____ and _____.
    A. Thought stopping, refuting irrational thoughts
    B. Meditation, progressive relaxation
    C. Therapeutic imagery, attention diversion
    D. Thought stopping, mediation

11. While rehabilitating an athlete you find he is excessively willing to do "whatever it takes" to recover fully and as quickly as possible. In doing so, you often have to remind the athlete not to push himself too hard and do too much. Which of the following is **not** a possible cause of overcompliance?
    A. Obsessive-compulsive behavior
    B. Slight feelings of denial
    C. Masking an underlying fear
    D. Manic-depressive behavior

12. During a football player's rehabilitation of a fractured lower leg, he will experience moments of intense pain. What may the athletic trainer suggest to the athlete as a means of controlling his own pain?
    A. Rehearse various plays in his mind
    B. Scream at the top of his lungs
    C. Tell the athletic trainer to stop when he feels a little discomfort
    D. Only come to therapy when no other athlete or coach is in the room

13. You notice after a severe wrist injury a gymnast you have been treating becomes sarcastic, loses her appetite, and appears unusually fatigued all the time. These are all symptoms of:
    A. Denial
    B. Anxiety
    C. Depression
    D. Anorexia

14. An athlete must be _____ and take _____ if he or she is to completely rehabilitate an injury.
    A. Emotionless, time off
    B. Passive, all prescribed medications
    C. Cooperative, responsibility
    D. Dependent, time off

15. Purging is a major symptom of:
    A. Bulimia
    B. Anorexia nervosa
    C. Obsessive-compulsive disorder
    D. Manic depression

16. Just before a big game, one of your athletes is demonstrating symptoms of moderate anxiety. Which of the following responses would be appropriate when caring for the athlete?
    A. Tell the athlete to "get a grip on himself"
    B. Tell the athlete you feel sorry for him
    C. Tell the athlete to talk to the coach
    D. Tell the athlete it is okay to be nervous but to focus on his goal

17. While treating an athlete for chronic patellar tendonitis, his coach tells you it is tough to get the athlete motivated to practice and his performance has significantly declined since the beginning of the season. What might the athletic trainer suspect the problem might be?
    A. Undertraining
    B. Staleness
    C. A personality disorder
    D. The athlete is accident-prone

18. An athlete who will be experiencing a long rehabilitation process and may have his position filled by another player may be at risk for which problem?
    A. Schizophrenia
    B. Mania
    C. Severe depression
    D. Bipolar disorder

19. What would be an appropriate action for the athletic trainer to take to relax an athlete who is very anxious about his injury?
    A. Teach the athlete about his injury
    B. Teach the athlete about controlled breathing
    C. Have the athlete speak with the school nurse
    D. Downplay the injury

20. An athlete is injured during an ice hockey game, and after being examined by the team physician is diagnosed with a complete anterior cruciate ligament tear. You have been told by the doctor this athlete cannot compete the rest of the season. When you see the athlete the next day he states, "The doctor doesn't know what he is talking about. I'll be fine." This athlete is demonstrating what behavior?
    A. Hysteria
    B. Depression
    C. Denial
    D. Bargaining

21. Which of the following actions taken by the athletic trainer can help make the athlete more compliant with rehabilitation of an injury?
    A. Have the coach threaten to kick him off the team if he does not cooperate
    B. Have the athlete bring a friend to the rehabilitation session
    C. Plan the rehabilitation sessions around the athlete's daily routine
    D. Make the rehabilitation sessions "fun"

22. Which of the following factors has a significant impact on the amount of stress an athlete will experience during his or her recovery from an injury?
    A. Whether or not soothing music is played in the training room
    B. Whether or not the coach is present during treatment
    C. Whether or not the same athletic trainer renders care
    D. The degree to which the athlete perceives he or she has control over his or her care

23. An athlete who wipes off his golf clubs after every shot and constantly makes sure it is returned to exactly the same spot in his bag every time it is used is demonstrating which of the following behaviors?
    A. Obsessive-compulsive
    B. Anxiety disorder
    C. Staleness
    D. Overachievement

24. Which of the following techniques allows the athlete to assess his or her own efforts at controlling a specific physiological response such as muscular tension?
    A. Moist heat pack
    B. Biofeedback
    C. Massage
    D. PNF

25. The anorexic female is usually a _____ and an _____.
    A. Hypochondriac, underachiever
    B. Perfectionist, overachiever
    C. Type B individual, underachiever
    D. Neurotic individual, anti-social personality

26. An athlete becomes hysterical after learning she has suffered a severe shoulder injury and cannot compete in her sport anymore. She is crying, screaming, and generally appears out of control. The appropriate response from the athletic trainer would be which of the following?
    A. Find her coach and have him deal with her
    B. Call her parents and have one of them calm her down
    C. Give the athlete "space"
    D. Allow the athlete to express her fears, but remain calm and demonstrate understanding. Assist the athlete in seeing the problem in proportion to the situation.

27. You have an athlete who comes to your office and is very depressed. He is not doing well academically, his parents are in the process of a divorce, and the coach just cut him from the baseball team after tryouts. He tells you he wants to kill himself. What is your appropriate response?
    A. Tell the athlete he should see a psychiastrist
    B. Listen to the athlete, take him seriously, and consult the team doctor immediately
    C. Tell the athlete he is not normal
    D. Ignore the athlete and hope the athlete will not do anything

Nutrition

1.   In which of the following foods is a high concentration of vitamin A found?
      A. Liver, yogurt, milk
      B. Red meat, oranges, tea
      C. Nuts, cereals, fish
      D. Liver, carrots, greens

2.   Vitamin C is also known as:
      A. Retinol
      B. Thiamin
      C. Ascorbic acid
      D. Niacin

3.   Besides sources such as fortified milk and fatty fish oils (such as in tuna fish), what is another major mode of obtaining vitamin D?
      A. Topical creams
      B. Sunlight
      C. Artichokes
      D. Fried beef liver

4.   The conversion of glucose to lactic acid is called:
      A. Photosynthesis
      B. Glycolysis
      C. Lactolysis
      D. The Krebs cycle

5.   When is the best time for an athlete to eat carbohydrate-rich foods?
      A. Within 2 hours after training
      B. 1 hour prior to training
      C. In small amounts while training
      D. A half-hour prior to training and throughout the training session

6.   At low workloads, muscle cells use _____ for fuel, while _____ is used for periods of intense exercise of short duration.
      A. Fat, protein
      B. Carbohydrate, fat
      C. Fat, phosphocreatine
      D. Protein, carbohydrate

7.   In which of the following foods would be a high concentration of the mineral phosphorus be found?
      A. Milk and cheese
      B. Dark green vegetables
      C. Oranges
      D. Table salt

8.   Which of the following are the "building blocks" of protein?
      A. Sugars
      B. Amino acids
      C. Triglycerides
      D. Sterols

9. The loss of _____ and _____ account for the greatest percentage of electrolytes lost through sweat.
   A. Potassium, chloride
   B. Magnesium, potassium
   C. Sodium, potassium
   D. Sodium, chloride

10. All of the following statements regarding fluid replacement during performance are appropriate **except**:
    A. The athlete should drink cold fluids to decrease body core temperature
    B. It is best for the athlete to consume small amounts of fluids frequently rather than large amounts of fluid infrequently
    C. Water is the ideal fluid replacement
    D. Do not force fluids on the athlete. He or she will seek out fluid replacement when thirsty.

11. Which of the categories below are **not** considered one of the six classes of nutrients?
    I.   Carbohydrates   IV. Water
    II. Proteins   V.   Fats
    III. Antioxidants   VI. Vitamins

    A. I, IV
    B. II, V
    C. V, VI
    D. III

12. Which of the following nutrients is absolutely necessary for every body chemical reaction to take place normally?
    A. Vitamins
    B. Amino acids
    C. Water
    D. Fats

13. Nutrition labels that are found on food packages allow the purchaser to compare nutritional values of food and are expressed in "percent daily values" (based on a 2000-calorie diet) that follow a new nutrient label, which used to be known as the US recommended daily allowance (US RDA). The new label now follows new standards known as:
    A. Recommended percent nutrients (RPN)
    B. US recommended daily allowances (US RDA)
    C. Reference daily intakes (RDI)
    D. US advised allowances (US AA)

14. All of the following are methods of measuring body composition **except**:
    A. Measuring muscle and fat girths
    B. Hydrostatic weighing
    C. Electrical impedance
    D. Measuring skin-fold thickness

15. Weight loss occurs when which of the following conditions exists?
    A. Less than 1000 calories are expended per day
    B. There is a negative caloric balance
    C. There is a positive caloric balance
    D. There is perfect caloric balance

16. Fat is a nutrient that is utilized as an energy source in the form of triglycerides. Triglycerides are stored in what type of cell?
    A. Striated
    B. Lypoma
    C. Beta
    D. Adipose

17. A football player desires to increase his body weight and wants to know how he should go about it in a safe manner. To increase his muscle mass without causing negative results, both his _____ and _____ should increase appropriately.
    A. Fat intake, carbohydrate intake
    B. Muscular exercise, dietary intake
    C. Dietary intake, caloric expenditure
    D. Caloric expenditure, water intake

18. One of your female cheerleaders has been diagnosed by your team physician with a combination of anorexia, osteoporosis, and amenorrhea. You recognize this combination as signs of:
    A. Marfan's syndrome
    B. The unhappy triad
    C. Female triad syndrome
    D. Paget's disease

19. One of your gymnasts has had a bone density test that has come back positive for mild osteoporosis. Which of the following minerals should be supplemented to prevent osteoporosis in a high-risk athlete?
    A. Calcium
    B. Niacin
    C. Folic acid
    D. Flouride

20. One of your male cross-county runners is a committed lactovegetarian. Which of the following minerals may be deficient with this type of diet?
    A. Calcium, flouride
    B. Iron, zinc
    C. Folic acid
    D. Copper, iron

21. One of your athletes goes out of his way to avoid eating carbohydrates such as bread and potatoes because of his fear of becoming fat. Which of the following substances will the body begin to utilize for energy if there is a significant lack of carbohydrates in the diet?
    A. Protein
    B. Fat
    C. Glucose
    D. Antioxidants

22. An athlete routinely complains of bloating, flatulence, and diarrhea after ingesting milk or ice cream. What might be the cause of this athlete's symptoms?
    A. Proteinuria
    B. Rickets
    C. Scurvy
    D. Lactase deficiency

23. Significant losses of electrolytes such as sodium, chloride, potassium, or magnesium during heavy exercise may lead to symptoms such as _____ or _____.
    A. Drop in pressure, diuresis
    B. Muscle strains, ligament strains
    C. Dyspnea, indigestion
    D. Muscular cramps, heat illness

24. Which two structures regulate water excretion?
    A. Kidneys, brain
    B. Kidneys, bladder
    C. Stomach, small intestines
    D. Kidneys, ureters

25. One of your baseball players reports he is having difficulty playing in the outfield under lights and has similar difficulty seeing at night while driving. While evaluating him you find out he hates vegetables and drinks milk infrequently. He "enjoys hamburgers and French fries." What substance might this athlete be lacking in his diet?
    A. Carbohydrates
    B. Protein
    C. Vitamin A
    D. Phosphorus

Pharmacology

1. Lomotil is what type of medication?
   A. Antibiotic
   B. Antidiarrheal
   C. Antifungal agent
   D. Antiemetic

2. Which of the following medications is often used for depression?
   A. Prozac
   B. Lithium
   C. Midol
   D. Ritalin

3. All of the following substances have stimulant properties **except**:
   A. Nicotine
   B. Theophylline
   C. Pseudephedrine
   D. Pepcid

4. Ibuprofen is available in which of the below dosages?
    I.   400 mg   IV. 50 mg
    II. 200 mg   V.   100 mg
    III. 600 mg   VI. 800 mg

    A. II, IV, V
    B. II, III, V
    C. III, V, VI
    D. I, II, III, VI

5. The brand name for the NSAID diclofenac is:
    A. Indocin
    B. Voltaren
    C. Orudis
    D. Feldene

6. What is the recommended dosage for the NSAID Naprosyn?
    A. 250 to 500 mg twice a day
    B. 500 to 750 mg twice a day
    C. 50 to 100 mg twice a day
    D. 200 mg once a day

7. Frequently abused drugs include stimulants such as amphetamines (speed), cocaine (coke or crack), and depressants (alcohol or downers). An athlete who has overdosed on a stimulant would manifest all of the following symptoms **except**:
    A. Agitation
    B. Decreased reaction time
    C. Rapid pulse and respirations
    D. Convulsions

8. Beta-blockers inhibit the action of catecholamines and decrease cardiac output. In which of the following sports would the effects of beta-blockers potentially enhance performance?
    A. Swimming
    B. Long-distance running
    C. Archery
    D. Baseball

9. In moderation, caffeine stimulates the _____ and _____ centers of the brain to cause increased alertness.
    A. Cerebral cortex, medulla
    B. Reticular formation, medulla
    C. Hypothalamus, midbrain
    D. Cerebellum, midbrain

10. The International Olympic Committee (IOC) divides performance-enhancing drugs into three classes. Class I drugs include which of the following?
    A. Blood reinjection (blood doping)
    B. Narcotics, diuretics, stimulants
    C. Alcohol, local anesthetics
    D. Narcotics, corticosteroids, alcohol

Physics

1. The area of the applicator that emits ultrasound that is expressed in square centimeters (cm^2) is known as:
   A. The transducer head surface area
   B. Effective emitting area
   C. Effective radiating area
   D. Direct-contact area

2. What is the frequency range of therapeutic ultrasound?
   A. 1.0 to 3.0 MHz
   B. 0.1 to 1 MHz
   C. 10,000 to 20,000 Hz
   D. 10,000 to 30,000 Hz

3. An object immersed in water experiences an upward force that is equal to the weight of the water displaced by the object. What law of physics is this?
   A. Archimedes' principle
   B. Wolf's law
   C. Pascal's law
   D. Bernoulli's law

4. A TENS unit is based on the _____ of pain control.
   A. Counter irritant theory
   B. Gate control theory
   C. Beta-endorphin theory
   D. Opiate theory

5. A pulsed current may be _____ or _____.
   A. Monophasic, biphasic
   B. Alternating, direct
   C. Direct, monophasic
   D. Alternating, biphasic

6. What is the most commonly used frequency in short-wave diathermy?
   A. 10 MHz
   B. 27.33 MHz
   C. 4068 Hz
   D. 2450 MHz

7. A modality that produces electromagnetic radiation with a frequency above 300 MHz and a wavelength shorter than 1 m is called:
    A. Infrared diathermy
    B. Short-wave diathermy
    C. Microwave diathermy
    D. Induction field diathermy

8. All of the following may be settings on a TENS unit **except**:
    A. Modulating
    B. Burst
    C. Continuous
    D. Surge

9. What kind of current is needed for iontophoresis?
    A. direct current
    B. Alternating current
    C. Alternating or direct current
    D. Ionized current

10. Which of the following is the correct definition of work?
    A. W = distance x velocity
    B. W = force x power
    C. W = force x distance
    D. W = pressure x distance

11. To perform iontophoresis, the medication used must be _____.
    A. Diluted
    B. Ionized
    C. In powder form
    D. Mixed with a gel

12. According to Joule's law, heat produced by high-frequency electrical currents is directly proportional to all of the following **except**:
    A. Power output
    B. Square of the current strength
    C. Resistance of the conductor
    D. Time during which the current flows

13. In the application of electrotherapy, the strength of an electrical current in a circuit is directly proportional to the applied electromotive force and inversely proportional to the resistance of the current. What law does this describe?
    A. Cosine law
    B. Ohm's law
    C. Joule's law
    D. Wolff's law

14. By what means does heat transfer to the skin with the use of a hot pack?
    A. Conduction
    B. Convection
    C. Radiation
    D. Evaporation

15. What type of waveform is produced when the current flow direction reverses on regular intervals?
    A. Galvanic current
    B. Pulsed current
    C. Alternating current
    D. Faradic current

16. The temperature of a thermometer reading is given in degrees Celsius. What formula must be used to convert the temperature from Celsius to Fahrenheit?
    A. (Temperature in Fahrenheit -32) x 5/9
    B. (Temperature in Celsius -32) x 5/9
    C. (Temperature in Celsius x 9/5) + 32
    D. (Temperature in Celsius + 32) x 5/9

17. What is the impedance of an electrical circuit?
    A. The pathway in which a current will flow
    B. The magnitude of the current flow
    C. The resistance within the circuit
    D. The direction of current flow

18. An athlete is evaluated by the athletic trainer and it is determined he has an acute supraspinatus tendinitis. Which of the following modalities is **not** appropriate to decrease pain and inflammation of the tendon?
    A. Phonophoresis
    B. Iontophoresis
    C. Moist heat packs
    D. Ice massage

19. The strength of a current flow is known as what?
    A. Rheobase
    B. Resistance
    C. Amperage
    D. Voltage

20. According to Poiseville's law, the _____ and _____ of a blood vessel is very critical in terms of resistance to blood flow.
    A. Length, radius
    B. Muscle type, contractility
    C. Length, thickness
    D. Direction, temperature

21. Which of the following intensities is considered medium intensity when treating an area with ultrasound?
    A. 0.8 to 1.5 watts per square cm
    B. 1.5 to 2.0 watts per square cm
    C. 1.0 to 3.0 total watts
    D. 5.0 to 8.0 total watts

22. How far from the skin surface should the ultrasound transducer head be kept when utilizing the underwater technique?
    A. Between 1 and 3 inches
    B. 3 inches
    C. 5 inches
    D. 0.5 to 1 inch from the skin surface

23. What is the polarity of an anode in an electrical stimulator?
    A. Disperse
    B. Negative
    C. Positive
    D. Neutral

Administration

1. Capital expenses of an athletic training program would include:
   A. Staff salaries
   B. Equipment under $500
   C. Athletic training supplies
   D. Buildings and room construction

2. A properly organized training room should have separate, designated areas for all the following **except**:
   A. Modality area
   B. Hydrotherapy area
   C. Storage facilities
   D. Changing room for the athletes

3. What is a practical, effective size for most school training rooms?
   A. 900 sq ft
   B. 1000 to 1200 sq ft
   C. 2000 to 3000 sq ft
   D. 800 to 1000 sq ft

4. How high should the electrical outlets be placed above the floor in the athletic training room?
   A. 2 to 3 ft
   B. 4 to 5 ft
   C. 6 ft
   D. 1 to 2 ft

5. Which of the following could present a problem for the athletic trainer when using a computer to store medical records?
    A. Maintaining security
    B. Retrieving specific informationl
    C. Loading files
    D. Using e-mail

6. How far from the nose should the face mask of a football helmet be located?
    A. 1 inch
    B. Two finger widths
    C. Three finger widths
    D. 0.75 inch

7. Thermomoldable plastics such as orthoplast or aquaplast may be indicated for many different situations. Which of the following conditions might benefit from the use of this type of material?
    A. Genu recurvatum
    B. Thoracic outlet syndrome
    C. Quadriceps contusion
    D. Anterior cruciate sprain

8. Which organization has identified the domains of athletic training as defined by the Role Delineation Study?
    A. AMA
    B. APTA
    C. NATABOC
    D. NATA Ethics Committee

9. Which of the following pieces of information are important for the athletic trainer to keep on record in the athletic training room?
    A. Injury reports
    B. Injury evaluations and progress notes
    C. Daily treatment logs
    D. All of the above

10. Which type of budget allocates a fixed amount of money for specific program functions and activities?
    A. Lump sum budgeting
    B. Fixed budgeting
    C. Line-item budgeting
    D. Variable budgeting

11. For a certified athletic trainer to maintain his or her certification by the NATABOC, how many continuing education units must he or she obtain in a 3-year period if he or she was certified before 1997?
    A. 60 CEUs
    B. 80 CEUs
    C. 20 CEUs
    D. 12 CEUs

12. Which of the following is the most restrictive form of regulation for the profession of athletic training?
    A. Exemption
    B. Certification
    C. Registration
    D. Licensure

13. To be a successful athletic trainer, an individual must possess all of the following personal qualities **except:**
    A. The ability to adapt to a changing environment
    B. A good sense of humor
    C. An interest in making money
    D. Empathy

14. Which of the following best describes the function of the school nurse in the sports medicine program of a high school?
    A. As a liaison between the athletic director and the athletic trainer
    B. The direct supervisor of the "health" services
    C. As the "first assistant" to the team physician
    D. As a liaison between the athletic trainer and the school health services

15. Which of the following organizations was established in 1950 and created a code of ethics and standards for the profession of athletic training?
    A. American Orthopaedic Society for Sports Medicine
    B. American College of Sports Medicine
    C. American Physical Therapy Association
    D. National Athletic Trainers' Association

Chapter IV

WRITTEN SIMULATION
SAMPLE QUESTIONS

A passing mark for <u>each section</u> of the following problems must be 80%. The passing mark is arrived by the number of correct responses encompassing 80% of the total number of questions per section. The authors recommend that if you do not pass a section at an 80% level, that you review the material that is relevant to that particular section.

Assign the appropriate value from the list identified below:

KEY
++ most appropriate answer
+ appropriate, but not first priority
0 no relevance to the problem
- not a priority/harmful
-- detrimental

For example: **Opening scene**: One of your wrestlers comes to the athletic training room complaining of a severe itching and burning sensation of the top of his scalp and he has noticed a lot of skin flaking with some hair loss.

Section A

How will you begin your evaluation of this athlete's condition? (Please select and prioritize your choices).

__ 1. Ask the athlete if he has had this problem before.
__ 2. Put gloves on and examine the athlete's scalp.
__ 3. Ask the athlete if he has had a recent cold.
__ 4. Administer an oral antibiotic medication from your athletic training kit.
__ 5. Use the athlete's teammate's towel to clean the area.

Correct answers to the above example:

Section A

The current situation: You know that your athlete has a dermatological problem.

Your immediate responsibility: To perform your initial evaluation to determine the type and extent of the problem.

1. +) It is appropriate to ask the athlete if he has had this problem before, because he may be able to provide you with important information regarding this condition.

2. ++) It is necessary and proper to don gloves and examine the athlete's scalp to determine the type and extent of this lesion.

3. 0) Asking the athlete if he has had a recent cold has no relevance to this problem.

4. --) It is not within the athletic trainer's scope of practice to administer a prescription drug without the direction of a supervising medical doctor.

5. -) This is an inappropriate action because this condition could be contagious and using another individual's towel is not sanitary.

Passing mark = 4 correct answers

PROBLEM I

Opening Scene

Two soccer players collide head-on during a game. You are called onto the field by the referee after your player does not get up off his back. You did not witness the collision.

Section A

How will you begin your initial evaluation of the athlete's condition? (Please select and prioritize your choices.)

___ 1. Ask the athlete where his pain is located.

___ 2. Immediately roll the athlete onto his side.

___ 3. Check to see if the athlete can move his fingers and toes.

___ 4. As you approach the field, ask any witnesses what occurred.

___ 5. Check the athlete for any areas that may be bleeding.

___ 6. Instruct a student athletic trainer to call for an ambulance.

___ 7. Evaluate the athlete's level of consciousness.

___ 8. Perform a primary survey.

___ 9. Ask the athlete if he has ever had a prior head injury.

___ 10. Note the position of the athlete.

___ 11. Ask if the athlete can stand and walk.

___ 12. Check the athlete's pupillary reactions with a penlight.

___ 13. Place an ice pack on the athlete's left shoulder

___ 14. Remove the athlete from the playing field.

___ 15. Ask the athlete if he can remember what happened and ask him to explain.

___ 16. Assess the athlete's pulse rate and blood pressure.

___ 17. Ask the student athletic trainer to go get a spine board.

___ 18. Sit the athlete up to make breathing easier.

Section B

The athlete is able to get up and walk off the field to the sidelines without assistance. Based on the information you now have, what would you do next? (Please select and prioritize your choices.)

___ 19. Perform a secondary survey.

___ 20. Ask the athlete if he knows where he is, if he knows the date, and what the name of his coach is.

___ 21. Escort the athlete to the training room and let him sleep.

___ 22. Give the athlete aspirin for a headache.

___ 23. Palpate the athlete's cervical area.

___ 24. Palpate the athlete's left upper trapezius muscle.

___ 25. Check the athlete's bilateral grip strength.

___ 26. Tell the coach the athlete is not to return to the game.

___ 27. Observe the athlete's posturing as he walks off the field.

___ 28. Note the athlete's skin color.

___ 29. Ask the athlete's parents what type of medical insurance they have.

___ 30. Call the team physician to gain guidance.

___ 31. Call the athlete's parents to make sure they arrange a doctor's visit the next day

___ 32. Elevate the athlete's feet.

___ 33. Give the athlete a pair of crutches.

Section C

Your athletic training staff has escorted the athlete to the training room. You meet the athlete there and reassess his injury. (Please select and prioritize your choices.)

___ 34. Record the athlete's vital signs every 10 minutes.

___ 35. Manually muscle test the upper trapezius muscle.

___ 36. Perform an Adson's test.

___ 37. Manually muscle test the deltoids.

___ 38. Manually muscle test the rotator cuff musculature.

___ 39. Have the athlete sit with his head between his knees.

___ 40. Have the athlete do a couple of deep squats.

___ 41. Ask the athlete to count backward from 50.

___ 42. Check the deep tendon reflex of the triceps bilaterally.

___ 43. Give the athlete oxygen by mask.

___ 44. Have the team physician come to the training room to reassess the injury.

___ 45. Have the athlete drive himself home.

___ 46. Check the athlete's sensation of the left upper arm.

___ 47. Check the active range of motion of the athlete's neck.

___ 48. Test for a Tinel's sign.

___ 49. Palpate the lateral epicondyle of the elbow for any tenderness.

___ 50. Manually muscle test the biceps.

___ 51. Manually muscle test the triceps.

Section D

The team physician as arrived and has re-evaluated the athlete. He determines the athlete has a first-degree concussion and a left-sided "burner." What would you do at this time? (Please select and prioritize your choices.)

___ 52. Put an ice pack on the athlete's left shoulder.

___ 53. Assess if the athlete still has sensory changes in his left upper arm or hand.

___ 54. Let the coach know the athlete has a minor injury and will play tomorrow.

___ 55. Have the physician write a note to keep the athlete home the next 2 days for observation by his parents.

___ 56. Give the athlete shoulder strengthening exercises.

___ 57. See if the athlete can do a few push-ups.

___ 58. Monitor the athlete the next few days for any changes in his condition.

___ 59. Make sure the team physician clears the athlete first before returning to play soccer.

___ 60. Give the athlete a soft neck collar to wear.

Problem II

Opening Scene

A wrestler from an opposing high school was elbowed in the nose prior to his arrival to your school for a county tournament. Throughout the tournament, he has been experiencing recurrent nosebleeds. He approaches you during an active nosebleed.

Section A

How will you begin your initial evaluation and treatment of the athlete's condition? (Please select and prioritize your choices.)

___ 1. Ask the athlete how hard he was hit.

___ 2. Ask the athlete if he has had a similar problem in the past.

___ 3. Ask the athlete if his parents are aware of his current problem.

___ 4. Ask the athlete if he has any allergies.

___ 5. Have the athlete put his head between his knees.

___ 6. Ask the athlete if he is dizzy.

___ 7. Take the athlete's pulse and blood pressure.

___ 8. Ask the athlete if his trainer has given him a noseguard.

___ 9. Place a warm compress on his nose.

___ 10. Ask the athlete if he has high blood pressure.

___ 11. Apply pressure to the athlete's right cheek.

___ 12. Palpate the athlete's nose and surrounding areas for pain and swelling.

___ 13. Observe the nose for swelling or deformity.

___ 14. Put an ice pack behind the athlete's neck.

___ 15. Allow the athlete to blow his nose to clear the nostril.

___ 16. Place a cotton nose plug under the athlete's top lip.

Section B

The nosebleed is beginning to stop. With this information, what would be your next steps? (Please select and prioritize your choices.)

___ 17. Perform a primary survey.

___ 18. Keep the athlete lying down with his legs elevated.

___ 19. Allow the athlete to apply finger pressure to the bridge of his nose.

___ 20. Allow your student trainer to find his coach or a responsible adult so your assessment can be shared.

___ 21. Do not let the athlete return to the competition for the rest of the day.

___ 22. Apply a nose splint.

___ 23. Have the athlete sit with his head tilted back.

__ 24. Call the athlete's home trainer.

__ 25. Use a cotton nose plug to stop the bleeding.

__ 26. Give the athlete aspirin for the swelling.

__ 27. Make sure there is no blood present on the athlete, his clothing, or the mat and floor.

Section C

The nosebleed has stopped. What would your final actions be and what instructions would you provide the athlete with at this time? (Please select and prioritize your choices.)

__ 28. Call your team doctor to report what happened.

__ 29. Call the athlete's team doctor to report what happened.

__ 30. Have the athlete's parents come to your training room.

__ 31. Limit the athlete's fluid intake.

__ 32. Allow the athlete to return to the competition.

__ 33. Send the athlete for x-rays.

__ 34. Call the athlete's athletic trainer to report what happened.

__ 35. Have the athlete do 10 sit-ups.

__ 36. Use a biohazard bag for any contaminated materials.

__ 37. Maintain close contact with the athlete during the remainder of the competition.

__ 38. Tell the athlete to keep an ice pack on his nose while he is not competing.

PROBLEM III

Opening Scene

A gymnast injures his right lower leg after a dismount off the rings. He appears to be in a lot of pain and has not stood up. He is lying on his left side. You did not witness this event.

Section A

How will you begin your initial evaluation of the athlete's condition? (Please select and prioritize your choices.)

__ 1. Ask the athlete what happened.

__ 2. Ask the athlete if he heard a snap.

__ 3. Check the right knee range of motion.

__ 4. Observe the leg for edema or bleeding.

__ 5. Palpate the leg for deformity.

__ 6. Check the athlete's vital signs.

__ 7. Palpate the athlete's popliteal pulse.

__ 8. Place a moist heat pack directly on the injury.

__ 9. Elevate the right leg.

__ 10. Have a coach call for an ambulance.

__ 11. Check the rest of body for any other injuries.

__ 12. Cut away the gymnast's pant leg (uniform).

__ 13. Immediately immobilize the lower right leg.

Section B

You have ruled out a compound fracture but suspect a fracture of both the tibia and fibula. With this information, how would you proceed at this time? (Please select and prioritize your choices.)

___ 14. If there is an obvious deformity of the bony shaft, try to reduce it to get good alignment.

___ 15. Remove the athlete from the mat to apply an immobilizer.

___ 16. Direct others to clear the area of people and equipment.

___ 17. Pack the right leg in ice.

___ 18. Check pulses in the ankle and foot.

___ 19. Check for Volkmann's contracture.

___ 20. Allow the competition to continue.

___ 21. Position the athlete in a supine position.

___ 22. Palpate the right hip joint.

___ 23. Elevate the entire leg.

___ 24. Check for crepitus.

___ 25. Immobilize the right lower leg.

___ 26. Massage the injured area.

Section C

The EMS team has arrived and the athlete is about to be transported to the emergency room. What are your final steps before he leaves with the EMS team? (Please select and prioritize your choices.)

___ 27. Check the lower extremity for numbness.

___ 28. Have the athlete walk to the ambulance with crutches.

___ 29. Issue NSAIDs for swelling.

___ 30. Have the coach follow the athlete to the hospital.

___ 31. Allow the athlete to eat and drink whatever he wants.

___ 32. Notify the coach that the athlete will no longer be permitted to participate for the rest of the season.

___ 33. Call ahead to the emergency room to make arrangements for his arrival.

___ 34. Check the athlete's symptoms of shock.

___ 35. Assure the athlete he will be taken care of before he departs.

___ 36. Fit the athlete for crutches.

___ 37. Call the athlete's parents.

___ 38. Fill out an injury report.

PROBLEM IV

Opening Scene

You are covering a basketball game when one of your players steps on another player's foot. You see the athlete twist his left ankle. He is jogging with an obvious limp. The coach calls a "time-out."

Section A

What will your initial evaluation include? (Please select and prioritize your choices.)

__ 1. Check the athlete's low back for an injury.

__ 2. Go get a wheelchair.

__ 3. Check the athlete's hamstring flexibility.

__ 4. Observe both ankles for swelling/deformity.

__ 5. Have the athlete jog off the court.

__ 6. Gently bang on the heel of the injured ankle.

__ 7. Perform a Lachman's test.

__ 8. Perform an anterior draw test on both ankles.

__ 9. Palpate the ankle and foot for areas of tenderness.

__ 10. Check the range of motion of the left ankle.

Section B

You have completed your initial evaluation and suspect that he has a second-degree lateral ankle sprain of his left ankle. With assistance, the athlete is brought into the training room. What is your initial treatment going to include? (Please select and prioritize your choices.)

__ 11. Keep the athlete in nonweight-bearing.

__ 12. Dispense aspirin to the athlete.

__ 13. Begin RICE

__ 14. Call the team doctor with your assessment.

__ 15. Begin ultrasound treatments.

__ 16. Place the left ankle in a hot whirlpool.

__ 17. Fit the athlete with crutches.

__ 18. Set up an appointment for an x-ray.

__ 19. Begin an upper body exercise program.

__ 20. After the game, present your findings to the coach.

__ 21. Begin a theraband strengthening program for the left ankle.

Section C

The team doctor is scheduled to be in the training room tomorrow morning. What instructions will you give the athlete for home? (Please select and prioritize your choices.)

__ 22. If he still has mild/moderate pain tonight, have the athlete go to the nearest emergency room.

__ 23. Call the athlete's parents with information on what happened.

__ 24. Begin lower extremity closed-chain exercises as tolerated.

__ 25. Keep ice packs on the ankle frequently and elevate it when the athlete is not ambulating.

__ 26. Keep a compression wrap on the ankle except when the athlete is sleeping.

__ 27. Have the athlete wear high-top sneakers.

__ 28. Have the athlete try to hop on the affected leg the next day to see if it still hurts.

PROBLEM V

Opening Scene

A field hockey player who is playing defense gets hit in the eye with a ball during a direct shot at the goal. She is lying on her side with her hands on her face.

Section A

How will you begin to evaluate the severity of the injury? (Please select and prioritize your choices.)

___ 1. Remove the face mask.

___ 2. Check that athlete's fine motor skills.

___ 3. Test the athlete's balance.

___ 4. Use an ammonia capsule to revive the athlete.

___ 5. Have the athlete walk off the field.

___ 6. Remove the mouthguard.

___ 7. Ask who made the shot.

___ 8. Ask the athlete where the pain is located.

___ 9. Palpate the athlete's shoulders.

___ 10. Perform a primary survey.

___ 11. Gently palpate the area around the orbit and nose for crepitus.

___ 12. Don latex gloves.

___ 13. Observe for a "battle sign."

___ 14. Ask the athlete if she is a scholarship athlete.

___ 15. Check the area for bleeding and lacerations.

___ 16. Ask the athlete if her vision is blurred.

Section B

The athlete has a deep laceration above the left eyebrow. Based on this information, what are your next steps? (Please select and prioritize your choices.)

___ 17. Check the pupil for reflex movements with a penlight.

___ 18. Apply moist heat to the eye.

___ 19. Rinse the wound with saline solution.

___ 20. Apply antiseptic ointment to the laceration.

___ 21. Cover both eyes with gauze pads.

___ 22. Have the athlete tell you what happened.

___ 23. Apply ice to the injury.

___ 24. Use Steri-strips to close the laceration.

___ 25. Ignore the athlete if she asks if there will be a scar.

___ 26. Use sutures to close the wound.

___ 27. Call for an ambulance.

___ 28. Have the athlete wait outside for the ambulance.

___ 29. Apply compression directly to the eye once you have "closed" the laceration.

___ 30. Perform a secondary survey.

Section C

You now have the laceration "closed" and are awaiting the ambulance. What are your final steps going to include? (Please select and prioritize your choices.)

___ 31. Keep the athlete calm.

___ 32. Announce the athlete's status over the public address system.

___ 33. Check the athlete's insurance plan.

___ 34. Call the school nurse to accompany the athlete to the hospital.

___ 35. Constantly change the bandage.

___ 36. Allow the athlete to speak to her coach.

___ 37. Allow the press access to the athlete.

___ 38. Wash your hands.

___ 39. Document the incident on an accident report form.

___ 40. Give the athlete a vitamin E pill.

___ 41. Report your findings and treatment plan to the athlete's coach.

PROBLEM VI

Opening Scene

The women's gymnastics coach reports to your office to discuss the behavior of one of her athletes. After reviewing what the coach has observed over the past month, you both suspect the athlete may be showing signs of anorexia nervosa.

Section A

With the information you now have available, how would you advise the coach to proceed? (Please select and prioritize your choices.)

___ 1. Confront the athlete with her problem and do not allow her to compete until the team physician examines her.

___ 2. Do not overemphasize the impact of lower body weight on the athlete's performance.

___ 3. Tell the coach to keep a diary of when the athlete eats.

___ 4. Have the coach encourage the athlete to maintain good nutritional habits to optimize her performance.

___ 5. Keep the athletic training staff informed if the athlete dramatically changes her behavior.

Section B

The athlete has talked with the coach and comes to your office to express her fear of being cut from the team. With the information available, how would you proceed? (Please select and prioritize your choices.)

___ 6. Assist the athlete in setting practical goals pertaining to safe means of dieting and determining a sensible target weight.

___ 7. Use "scare" tactics to discourage the use of laxatives and diuretics.

___ 8. Encourage the athlete to express her fears and concerns regarding her weight and athletic abilities.

___ 9. Address the issue with your athletic director.

___ 10. Discuss the athlete's options in case she is cut from the gymnastics team.

___ 11. Tell the athlete she has nothing to worry about and you will talk to the coach for her.

___ 12. Tell the athlete she should think about getting professional counseling to overcome her problem.

___ 13. Set up a meeting between the coach, athlete, and yourself to discuss what has been observed and how it will be managed.

Section C

The athlete concedes to the coach and the athletic trainer that she may have an eating disorder. With this information available, what are your next steps? (Please select and prioritze your choices.)

___ 14. Call your team physician.

___ 15. Set up an appointment with a psychologist.

___ 16. Put the athlete on a strict diet emphasizing weight gain.

___ 17. Weigh the athlete on a daily basis.

___ 18. Arrange for the athlete to be hospitalized for a week to force feed her.

___ 19. Arrange counseling meetings for the athlete with a sports nutritionist.

___ 20. Put the athlete on a diet consisting of Ensure, bananas, and red meat at least twice a day.

PROBLEM VII

Opening Scene

While covering a state track meet, you observe a high jumper land incorrectly on the crash mat. When you get to the high jump pit, you see him lying on his right side and he is not moving.

Section A

Given the above information, what would your initial steps be in evaluating the condition of this athlete? (Please select and prioritize your choices.)

___ 1. Call for an ambulance.

___ 2. Ask the athlete where he has pain.

___ 3. Do a primary survey.

___ 4. Make a mental note as to how the athlete is positioned.

___ 5. With assistance from a student trainer, turn the athlete onto his back.

___ 6. Ask the athlete to wiggle his fingers and toes.

___ 7. Ask the athlete what occurred.

___ 8. Place an ice pack on the athlete's neck.

___ 9. Palpate the athlete's knees for deformity.

___ 10. Check the athlete for any areas of bleeding on his face.

___ 11. Send for the athlete's parents.

___ 12. Check the athlete's level of consciousness.

Section B

After speaking to the athlete and completing your initial evaluation, you suspect a potentially serious neck injury. What would your next steps be in caring for this athlete? (Please select and prioritze your choices.)

___ 13. With assistance, carry the athlete to the sidelines.

___ 14. To determine the severity of the injury, see if the athlete can rotate his head.

___ 15. Ask the athlete if he has any numbness or tingling down either upper extremity.

___ 16. Tell the athlete not to try to move his head.

___ 17. Check the athlete's pupillary response with a penlight.

___ 18. Do a check of cranial nerves IV through XII.

___ 19. With assistance of at least two to four other people and while maintaining the head in neutral, log-roll the athlete into a supine position.

___ 20. Ask the officials to stop the meet.

___ 21. Secure the athlete on a spine board.

___ 22. Ask someone to call an ambulance.

___ 23. Place the athlete in a cervical collar.

___ 24. Monitor the athlete's vital signs.

Section C

The athlete is brought by ambulance to the hospital. What would your next actions be? (Please select and prioritize your choices.)

___ 25. Contact your team physician.

___ 26. Fill out an accident report form.

___ 27. Return to the meet and follow-up with the athlete at a later time.

___ 28. Check your records to see if the athlete is allergic to any medications.

___ 29. Check with the coach to see if the athlete is on a scholarship.

___ 30. Contact the athlete's parents to inform them of the accident.

___ 31. Follow the ambulance to the hospital and leave your senior student trainer to cover the meet.

___ 32. Suggest to the athletic director that the school should eliminate the high jump event next time because it is too dangerous.

PROBLEM VIII

Opening Scene

One of your female cross-country runners comes into the athletic training room complaining of chronic left anterior knee pain, which comes and goes with activity.

Section A

Your initial evaluation of this problem would include which of the following actions? (Please select and prioritize your choices.)

___ 1. Put an ice pack on the athlete's knee.

___ 2. Observe the athlete's posture.

___ 3. Palpate the anteromedial joint line for tenderness and swelling.

___ 4. Perform a bilateral Ober's test.

___ 5. Ask the athlete if she feels a popping sensation while walking or running.

___ 6. Ask the athlete if she has ever injured her foot before.

___ 7. Perform a Patrick's test.

___ 8. Ask the athlete if the knee hurts going up and down stairs.

___ 9. Tell the athlete to stop running when it hurts.

___ 10. See how the athlete responds to temporary orthotics.

___ 11. Observe the left knee for swelling.

___ 12. Palpate the patellar area for tenderness.

___ 13. Perform a KT-1000 test.

Section B

After your initial evaluation, you conclude this athlete has a chronically subluxing patella. What steps would you take at this time to treat this athlete? (Please select and prioritze your choices.)

___ 14. Recommend the athlete wear a soft brace to stabilize the patella during running.

___ 15. Teach the athlete exercises to strengthen her hamstrings.

___ 16. Teach the athlete exercises to strengthen her left VMO.

___ 17. Tell the athlete to perform deep squatting exercises two to three times per day.

___ 18. Evaluate the effect of patellar taping with activity.

___ 19. Teach the athlete iliotibial band stretching exercises.

___ 20. Tell the athlete to consistently stretch her hamstrings.

___ 21. Give the athlete Voltaren.

___ 22. Tell the athlete to avoid soft, flat surfaces while running.

Section C

To speed up this athlete's rehabilitation, you decide she should come to see you on a daily basis for treatment in the training room. Which activities/treatments would you perform for this condition? (Please select and prioritze your choices.)

___ 23. Apply a TENS unit to the left knee for pain.

___ 24. Perform PNF exercises, which emphasize hip flexion, abduction, and internal rotation.

___ 25. Apply ultrasound treatments to promote healing.

___ 26. Instruct the athlete in plyometric activities.

___ 27. Have the athlete perform both open- and closed-chain quadriceps exercises.

___ 28. Evaluate the athlete's running gait on a treadmill.

___ 29. Have the athlete perform exercises that strengthen the hip adductors.

___ 30. Routinely apply ice packs to the affected knee after activity.

PROBLEM IX

Opening Scene

You are traveling with your school's men's basketball team when one of your athletes comes to you complaining he has been having abdominal cramping and intermittent diarrhea for the past 2 days.

Section A

Based on the above information, how would you proceed with your initial assessment for this athlete? (Please select and prioritize your choices.)

___ 1. Ask the athlete what his diet has consisted of (food and drink) during the past 2 to 3 days.

___ 2. Ask the athlete if he is nervous about playing.

___ 3. Ask the athlete if he has had this problem before.

___ 4. Check the athlete's blood pressure.

___ 5. Take the athlete's oral temperature.

___ 6. Check the athlete's body fat levels.

___ 7. Palpate the athlete's abdomen.

___ 8. Have the athlete run on a treadmill for 20 minutes.

Section B

Assuming from your evaluation that this athlete has a gastrointestinal upset because of precompetition anxiety, what might your next steps be in assisting in this athlete's recovery? (Please select and prioritize your choices.)

__ 9. Speak with the coach and have the athlete refrain from practice until the symptoms disappear.

__ 10. Weigh the athlete before and after practices and games.

__ 11. Give the athlete antimotility drugs such as Imodium.

__ 12. Make sure the athlete eats a lot of green vegetables like broccoli and cabbage.

__ 13. Give the athlete milk, soda, or tea to rehydrate.

__ 14. Buy a water-testing kit and evaluate the hotel's drinking water.

__ 15. Have the athlete only drink bottled water.

PROBLEM X

Opening Scene

A soccer player injures his knee during practice. He is assisted into the training room by two teammates. Upon your initial observation, you notice he is limping and his right knee is visibly swollen.

Section A

Given the above information, how would you proceed with your initial evaluation of this athlete? (Please select and prioritize your choices.)

__ 1. Palpate the knee joint and surrounding areas for point tenderness.

__ 2. Ask the athlete if he can do a deep squat without pain.

__ 3. Ask the athlete what happened.

__ 4. Check the dorsalis pedis pulse of the affected limb.

__ 5. Ask the athlete if he heard or felt a snap or pop.

__ 6. Perform a Speed's test.

__ 7. Perform a Lachman's test.

__ 8. Check the knee for crepitus.

__ 9. Ask the athlete if he has had a prior injury to the affected knee.

__ 10. Measure the range of motion of the affected knee.

__ 11. Assess the strength of the athlete's hip abductors.

__ 12. Ask the athlete to perform toe raises.

__ 13. Perform a pivot shift test on the involved knee.

Section B

After evaluating the athlete's knee, you suspect the athlete has injured his anterior cruciate ligament. What steps would you take at this time? (Please select and prioritize your choices.)

__ 14. Issue crutches to the athlete and instruct him in toe-touch weightbearing.

__ 15. Wrap the athlete's knee in ice and elevate his leg.

__ 16. Call the team physician.

__ 17. Apply McConnell taping to the injured knee.

___ 18. Instruct the athlete to use a heating pad on his knee when he is at rest at home.

___ 19. Order a functional brace for use during activity.

___ 20. Apply ultrasound (pulsed) to the injured knee.

Section C

The team physician comes to the training room and, after examining the athlete, agrees with your assessment and recommends the athlete have an MRI to confirm the physical findings. Until the severity of the injury is known, he asks you to instruct the athlete in the appropriate treatments for home. (Please select and prioritize your choices.)

___ 21. Instruct the athlete in knee and hip active range of motion exercises as tolerated.

___ 22. Have the athlete apply ice to the knee every few hours to minimize swelling.

___ 23. Tell the athlete to wean himself from the crutches to a cane over the next 24 hours.

___ 24. Work on proprioception by having the athlete practice balancing on the unaffected leg twice a day.

___ 25. Instruct the athlete to perform isometric quadriceps and hamstring exercises.

___ 26. Give the athlete a TENS unit for home use.

___ 27. Have the athlete practice going up and down stairs and jog as normally as possible.

Problem XI

Opening Scene

A football player comes to you requesting help in improving his general lower body strength and overall conditioning.

Section A

What suggestions would you make in assisting this athlete in a preseason training program? (Please select and prioritize your choices.)

___ 1. Give the athlete anabolic steroids.

___ 2. Instruct the athlete in a general flexibility program.

___ 3. Have the athlete run up and down the stadium stairs in pads.

___ 4. Monitor the athlete's respiratory rate while at rest.

___ 5. Incorporate warm-up and cool-down periods.

___ 6. Make the exercises sport-specific.

___ 7. Have the athlete participate in other sports such as basketball or tennis.

___ 8. Have the athlete perform progressive-resistance lower extremity exercises 3 days a week.

___ 9. Put the athlete on a red meat and legume diet.

___ 10. Mix up the training schedule to keep it interesting.

___ 11. Keep the training schedule intense and emphasize training for long periods of time (eg, 3 to 4 hours).

___ 12. Progress the conditioning program gradually as the athlete improves his tolerance for work.

___ 13. Help the athlete adjust to working in the heat.

Section B

As the football season begins, the athlete continues to seek your advice to keep him fit and healthy. What types of things might you emphasize to keep him in condition during the season? (Please select and prioritize your choices.)

___ 14. Have the athlete run 2 miles three times a week.

___ 15. Continue strength training exercises for the lower body.

___ 16. Make sure the athlete takes 2 to 3 days off a week so he gets adequate rest.

___ 17. Monitor the athlete's blood pressure on a daily basis.

___ 18. Have the athlete perform plyometric activities for power.

___ 19. Establish a maintenance-conditioning program to be performed on a regular basis.

___ 20. Put the athlete on a clear liquid diet.

___ 21. Have the athlete participate in a cross-training program.

___ 22. Give the athlete a tennis ball to work on grip strengthening.

___ 23. Encourage the athlete to take a class in Judo.

Section C

What types of activities might you suggest the athlete participate in as part of an off-season program? (Please select and prioritize your choices.)

___ 24. Continue a general flexibility program.

___ 25. Have the athlete participate in a cross-training program.

___ 26. Have the athlete jog four to five times a week.

___ 27. Have the athlete eat a high-calorie diet to build up muscle strength.

___ 28. Have the athlete meet with a sport psychologist to learn visual imagery.

___ 29. No physical activity. This is the period during which the athlete should rest and recover.

___ 30. Give the athlete time during his training schedule to participate in nonathletic events.

___ 31. Have the athlete take up another sport to stay in shape.

PROBLEM XII

Opening Scene

An ice hockey player slams head-first into the boards during practice. He is lying face down on the ice and is not moving. You have witnessed this event and no other players are involved.

Section A

How will you begin your initial evaluation of this athlete's condition? (Please select and prioritize your choices.)

___ 1. Perform a secondary survey of the athlete's entire body.

___ 2. With assistance, roll the athlete onto his back while maintaining the head and neck in neutral.

___ 3. Remove the athlete's helmet.

___ 4. Perform a primary survey.

___ 5. Establish the level of consciousness.

___ 6. Begin chest compressions.

___ 7. Have the coach get a vacu-splint.

___ 8. Ask the other players what happened during the last play.

___ 9. Sit the athlete up so he can breathe.

Section B

You have determined the athlete is unconscious and is not breathing, but he has a pulse. What are your next steps in treating this athlete? (Please select and prioritize your choices.)

___ 10. Perform a secondary survey.

___ 11. Have the coach call for an ambulance.

___ 12. Vigorously shake the athlete to try and get a response.

___ 13. Take the athlete's blood pressure.

___ 14. Cut off the face mask.

___ 15. Log-roll the athlete onto his side.

___ 16. Check the athlete for a positive Romberg's sign.

___ 17. Perform abdominal thrusts to clear the airway.

___ 18. Begin artificial respiration.

___ 19. Establish if the athlete is in cardiac arrest.

___ 20. Remove the athlete's mouthguard.

___ 21. Use a jaw-thrust to open the athlete's airway.

Section C

The EMS team has arrived. The athlete begins breathing again and becomes responsive. He states he cannot feel anything. With this information, what will be your next actions? (Please select and prioritize your choices.)

___ 22. Perform a secondary survey.

___ 23. Continue to monitor breathing, pulse, and blood pressure.

___ 24. Tell the athlete not to worry, that he should feel something soon, and it is a temporary problem.

___ 25. With assistance, secure the athlete onto a spine board while maintaining the head and neck in neutral.

___ 26. Call your team doctor.

___ 27. Check pupillary response with a penlight.

___ 28. Argue with the EMS team about whether or not the athlete's helmet should be removed.

___ 29. Tell the coach you will be at the emergency room and you will be in touch with him later.

___ 30. Fill out an incident report to document what happened.

Section D

After practice, you go to the hospital to check on the athlete's condition. The emergency room physician informs you the athlete will probably be a C5-6 quadriplegic. With this information available, what would you do next? (Please select and prioritize your choices.)

___ 31. Check on the athlete to see how he is doing.

___ 32. Call the team physician to inform him what has happened.

___ 33. Contact the athlete's parents.

___ 34. Tell the athlete sometimes doctors make mistakes and not to give up hope.

___ 35. Check your liability insurance.

___ 36. Call the local newspaper to give them the story.

___ 37. Return to school and inform the coach.

___ 38. With the coaching staff, inform the team what has happened.

___ 39. Have the emergency room physician contact your athletic director.

PROBLEM XIII

Opening Scene

The pitcher from your baseball team comes to the training room with complaints of a deep ache in his right shoulder which occurs after pitching and lingers for a number of hours after he stops the activity. He also states his right arm feels unusually fatigued after throwing a short period of time. He reports his shoulder feels the best when he has his right hand in his pants pocket. You have seen him voluntarily sublux his shoulders in the past as he was telling his friends he is double-jointed.

Section A

What questions would be appropriate to ask during the history portion of your initial exam? (Please select and prioritize your choices.)

___ 1. Ask the athlete how long he has had this problem.

___ 2. Ask the athlete when the last time his right shoulder was injured.

___ 3. Ask the athlete what specific actions/positions make the pain worse.

___ 4. Ask the athlete if he is eating enough protein.

___ 5. Ask the athlete if his shoulder feels like it slips with activity.

___ 6. Ask the athlete if he is double-jointed.

___ 7. Ask the athlete if he is taking his vitamins.

___ 8. Ask the athlete what the intensity of the pain is on a scale of 0 to 10. (0 representing no pain, 10 representing excruciating pain).

___ 9. Ask the athlete if his father had the same problem when he played baseball.

___ 10. Ask the athlete if he is taking any medications for the pain.

Section B

With the information obtained from the history, which of the following special tests would be appropriate when examining this shoulder? (Please select and prioritize your choices.)

___ 11. Phalen's test.

___ 12. Clunk test.

___ 13. Pivot shift test.

___ 14. Patrick's test.

___ 15. Thompson test.

___ 16. Apprehension test (anterior and posterior).

___ 17. Hawkins-Kennedy test.

___ 18. Neer sign.

___ 19. Posterior drawer test (of the shoulder).

___ 20. Ober test.

___ 21. Trendelenburg test.

___ 22. Sulcus sign.

Section C

After completing your evaluation, you suspect the athlete has multidirectional instability of the right shoulder. Knowing what you do about this condition, which of the following exercises would be appropriate to specifically strengthen the scapular stabilizers and rotator cuff musculature? (Please select and prioritize your choices.)

___ 23. Shoulder shrugs.

___ 24. Biceps curls.

___ 25. Shoulder abduction exercises with free weights.

___ 26. Cervical isometric exercises.

___ 27. Internal/external rotation of the shoulder using theraband.

___ 28. Manual PNF exercises (D2 extension pattern).

___ 29. Triceps curls.

___ 30. Rowing exercises.

___ 31. Serratus anterior strengthening exercises.

___ 32. Partial sit-ups.

___ 33. Prone trunk extensions.

___ 34. Calf raises.

PROBLEM XIV

Opening Scene

You are covering a tennis match when one player runs to the net for a volley, stops and sets for the shot, and suddenly falls to the court while grabbing his left lower leg. He is in severe pain.

Section A

With the information you have available, how will you begin your initial evaluation of this injury? (Please select and prioritize your choices.)

___ 1. Establish if the athlete is breathing.

___ 2. Ask the athlete to walk off the court.

___ 3. Ask the athlete what happened.

___ 4. Determine the athlete's level of consciousness according to the Glasgow Coma Scale.

___ 5. Check the athlete's leg for bleeding.

___ 6. Ask the athlete where the pain is located.

___ 7. Observe the left lower extremity for any deformity

___ 8. Ask the athlete if he felt a snap or pop.

___ 9. Have a student trainer apply an ice bag to the leg.

___ 10. Ask the athlete if he has ever injured his right leg before.

___ 11. Ask the athlete if he can hop on the left leg.

Section B

You assist the athlete off the court and have him sit on a bench. What actions would you perform at this time? (Please select and prioritize your choices.)

___ 12. Palpate the calf for pain, swelling, or deformity.

___ 13. Perform a Lachman's test bilaterally.

___ 14. Perform a Thomas test bilaterally.

___ 15. Check active range of motion of both ankles.

___ 16. Measure the Q-angle of the right leg.

__ 17. Check to see if the athlete has bunions.

__ 18. Perform a Thompson test bilaterally.

__ 19. Perform a Hawkin's test bilaterally.

__ 20. Perform an anterior drawer test bilaterally on both ankles.

__ 21. Palpate the left femoral pulse.

__ 22. Test the patellar tendon reflex bilaterally.

__ 23. Manually muscle test the ankle plantar flexors bilaterally.

Section C

Based on your initial assessment, you determine the athlete has a torn gastrocnemius muscle. The athlete is transported to the training room in a golf cart. What would your initial treatment consist of during week 1? (Please select and prioritize your choices.)

__ 24. Warm whirlpool treatments.

__ 25. Applying ice packs to the lower leg.

__ 26. Applying a compression wrap.

__ 27. High volt galvanic stimulation.

__ 28. Posterior lower leg splint.

__ 29. Range of motion exercises on the BAPS board.

__ 30. Calf raises.

__ 31. Fitting the athlete with crutches.

__ 32. Applying an antibiotic ointment to the defect.

__ 33. Begin hamstring curls with weight.

__ 34. Start ultrasound treatments.

__ 35. Begin gentle active range of motion exercises for the right ankle.

Section D

Four weeks have passed since the initial injury. The athlete has minimal/no discomfort with active plantar flexion, but the movement is still weak against resistance (4/5). All other ankle and knee motions are within normal ranges. Which of the following exercises would be appropriate? (Please select and prioritize your choices.)

__ 36. Stationary bike.

__ 37. Uphill jogging.

__ 38. Push-ups.

__ 39. Progressive-resistance ankle exercises.

__ 40. Plyometric exercises.

__ 41. Upper body ergometer.

__ 42. Proprioception exercises.

__ 43. Calf raises.

__ 44. Partial squats.

__ 45. Progressive-resistance hamstring exercises.

__ 46. Progressive-resistance quadriceps exercises.

__ 47. General lower extremity flexibility exercises.

__ 48. Biceps curls.

__ 49. Shoulder press.

__50. Agility exercises.

Section E

Six weeks have passed since the initial injury. The athlete has done very well during his rehabilitation. What specific criteria would you use to determine that this athlete is fully recovered and ready to participate in tennis? (Please select and prioritize your choices.)

___ 51. The athlete can walk 50 feet without a limp.

___ 52. The athlete has no complaints of lower extremity pain at rest or during activity.

___ 53. There is no visible swelling or ecchymosis.

___ 54. There is no pain with palpation of the injured area.

___ 55. The athlete has no pain while performing a hamstring curl.

___ 56. The athlete has full ankle and knee range of motion.

___ 57. The coach demands the athlete's return to competition.

___ 58. The athlete can hop on the injured leg without pain.

___ 59. The athlete can jog on the treadmill for 20 minutes without pain.

___ 60. The athlete is getting bored with his rehabilitation program.

___ 61. The strength of the athlete's left ankle and leg is equal to the right side.

___ 62. The team physician clears the athlete to return to full activity.

___ 63. The athlete can bench press 50 pounds or more.

PROBLEM XV

Opening Scene

A wrestler stops by the training room after practice complaining of chronic low back pain which increases a few hours to a day after a workout. He states he has had this pain before and has seen an orthopaedic surgeon who had diagnosed him with a chronic low back strain. The athlete denies having any radicular signs and states the pain is localized to the lumbar area.

Section A

With the information that is available to you, what would your initial evaluation include? (Please select and prioritize your choices.)

___ 1. Observe the athlete's posture in standing.

___ 2. Ask the athlete to describe his pain.

___ 3. Check the range of motion of both knees.

___ 4. Perform a Scour test of the right hip.

___ 5. Palpate the lumbar erector spinae.

___ 6. Observe the low back for signs of atrophy.

___ 7. Palpate the PSIS bilaterally.

___ 8. Check the athlete for genu varum.

___ 9. Check the athlete for a leg-length discrepancy.

___ 10. Have the athlete do a partial squat.

___ 11. Evaluate the range of motion of the lumbar spine.

___ 12. Measure hip abduction with a goniometer.

___ 13. Check the flexibility of the hamstrings and hip flexors.

Section B

Your findings from the initial evaluation are consistent with a chronic lumbar strain. The athlete does not appear to be in severe pain but does seem uncomfortable with active lumbar movement. Which of the following modalities would be appropriate to decrease this athlete's pain? (Please select and prioritize your choices.)

__ 14. Friction massage.

__ 15. Ice packs.

__ 16. Warm whirlpool treatments (full body).

__ 17. Ultrasound.

__ 18. Iontophoresis.

__ 19. Ice massage.

__ 20. Chiropractic treatments.

__ 21. TENS therapy.

__ 22. Moist heat packs.

__ 23. Short-wave diathermy.

__ 24. Stationary bicycling.

__ 25. Functional electric stimulation.

__ 26. Cervical traction.

__ 27. Paraffin bath.

__ 28. Effleurage.

__ 29. Neoprene lumbar support.

Section C

Regarding the initial phases (I and II) of the rehabilitation program, which of the following exercises would be most appropriate? (Please select and prioritize your choices.)

__ 30. Active trunk extensions in prone.

__ 31. Gentle active assisted low back stretching.

__ 32. Resisted knee extensions.

__ 33. Passive hamstring stretching.

__ 34. Active posterior pelvic tilts.

__ 35. Passive iliopsoas stretching.

__ 36. PNF exercises to the hip and lower extremity.

__ 37. Lower trunk rotations in supine.

Section D

Regarding the later phases (III and IV) of the rehabilitation program, which of the following exercises would be most appropriate? (Please select and prioritize your choices.)

__ 38. PNF exercises to the trunk.

__ 39. Resistive abdominal strengthening.

__ 40. Resistive cervical strengthening.

__ 41. Resistive prone hip extension.

__ 42. Achilles stretching exercises.

__ 43. Groin stretching exercises.

__ 44. Shoulder press.

__ 45. Jogging.

__ 46. Swimming.

__ 47. Resistive bridging exercises.

__ 48. Trunk extensions in prone.

PROBLEM XVI

Opening Scene

One of your swimmers comes to your office complaining of severe ear pain that is accompanied by intense itching and a mild discharge.

Section A

Upon examining the athlete's ear, you notice the ear canal is inflamed and the athlete has partial hearing loss. Based on these findings, you determine the athlete has external otitis (swimmer's ear). What should you do to begin treatment of this condition? (Please select and prioritize your choices.)

__ 1. Dispense penicillin.

__ 2. Clear out the ear with a Q-tip soaked in epinephrine.

__ 3. Arrange for the athlete to see the team physician.

__ 4. Cover the ear with a sterile gauze pad.

__ 5. Advise the athlete to wear a hood in cold environments.

__ 6. Use a TENS unit for pain.

__ 7. Apply a moist heat pack to the affected ear.

__ 8. Allow the athlete to continue swimming as tolerated.

Section B

The team physician comes to the athletic training room, examines the athlete, and makes a diagnosis of external otitis. He dispenses an oral antibiotic and ear drops (3% boric acid and alcohol) to be administered daily. In addition to these treatments, you instruct the athlete in which of the following measures? (Please select and prioritize your choices.)

__ 9.   Protect the athlete's ear while swimming with a plug of lamb's wool soaked with lanolin.

__ 10. Have the athlete wear a bathing cap when swimming.

__ 11. Have the athlete cross-train to prevent frustration from not swimming.

__ 12. Instruct the athlete to wear goggles while swimming.

__ 13. Instruct the athlete not to stick any object into his ears.

PROBLEM XVII

Opening Scene

You are covering a men's varsity basketball game when one of your players is observed injuring his right knee while rebounding a ball. He is able to limp off the court unassisted. He reports his knee bent sideways when he landed. He states he felt a sharp pain, but cannot recall feeling a pop or snap.

Section A

What actions would you take during your initial assessment of this injury? (Please select and prioritize your choices.)

__ 1. Ask the athlete to point to where he feels pain.

__ 2. Observe the right knee for swelling or deformity.

__ 3. Apply an ice pack to the knee.

__ 4. Apply a knee immobilizer to the injured extremity.

__ 5. Issue a cane to the athlete.

__ 6. Palpate the right knee anterolateral/anteromedial joint line.

__ 7. Palpate the right gluteus medius muscle.

__ 8. Have the athlete perform 10 calf raises.

__ 9. Check the range of motion of both knee joints.

__ 10. Ask the athlete if he has ever injured his right knee before.

__ 11. Manually muscle test the strength of the hip flexors bilaterally.

__ 12. Manually muscle test the strength of the quadriceps bilaterally.

__ 13. Manually muscle test the strength of the hamstrings bilaterally.

__ 14. Check the athlete's pupillary reaction.

Section B

What special tests would you perform during your evaluation of this injury? (Please select and prioritize your choices.)

__ 15. Lachman's test bilaterally.

__ 16. Vertebral artery test bilaterally.

__ 17. Tinel's test bilaterally.

__ 18. Valgus stress test bilaterally.

__ 19. Varus stress test bilaterally.

__ 20. Posterior drawer test bilaterally.

__ 21. Empty can test bilaterally.

__ 22. Finkelstein test bilaterally.

__ 23. Yergason's test bilaterally.

__ 24. McMurray test bilaterally.

__ 25. Anterior drawer test bilaterally.

__ 26. Pivot shift test bilaterally.

__ 27. Patellar apprehension test bilaterally.

Section C

After being examined by the team physician, the athlete is diagnosed with a second-degree medial collateral sprain. What actions would you take to control the pain and swelling and address the limitations in range of motion? (Please select and prioritize your choices.)

__ 28. Apply moist heat packs to the right knee.

__ 29. Massage the knee joint.

__ 30. Have the athlete use a rowing machine.

__ 31. Fit the athlete with crutches.

___ 32. Manually muscle test the quadriceps.

___ 33. Begin isotonic hamstring strength exercises.

___ 34. Apply ice packs to the knee.

___ 35. Have the athlete perform active knee extension and flexion range of motion exercises as tolerated.

___ 36. Have the athlete elevate his left leg during the course of the day.

___ 37. Give the athlete Tylenol with codeine for pain.

___ 38. Use high volt galvanic stimulation.

Section D

The team physician recommends the athlete begin rehabilitation in 1 week. Knowing the athlete will be unable to return to basketball for approximately 4 to 5 weeks, how would you go about beginning a functional exercise program and maintain his aerobic condition during weeks 1 to 2 post-injury? (Please select and prioritize your choices.)

___ 39. Swimming (regular crawl).

___ 40. Calf raises.

___ 41. Running on the treadmill.

___ 42. Stairmaster (low resistance).

___ 43. Upper body ergometer.

___ 44. Wall pulley exercises (upper extremity).

___ 45. Stationary bicycling.

___ 46. Fartlek training.

___ 47. Plyometric exercises.

___ 48. Rowing machine.

Problem XVIII

Opening Scene

A soccer player jumps up to head a ball. While he is in the air, he is kicked in the abdominal area by an opponent. He curls up in pain on the ground.

Section A

What steps would you take during your initial evaluation of this athlete? (Please select and prioritize your choices.)

___ 1. Perform a primary survey.

___ 2. Give the athlete oxygen.

___ 3. Auscultate the athlete's heart.

___ 4. Palpate the abdominal area.

___ 5. Ask the athlete where the pain is located.

___ 6. Have the athlete stand and jog a little.

___ 7. Have the athlete count backward from 100.

___ 8. Have a student athletic trainer bring out a stretcher.

___ 9. Put on a latex glove before touching the athlete.

___ 10. Observe the abdominal area for edema or ecchymosis.

___ 11. Ask if the pain radiates anywhere.

Section B

Following your initial evaluation, you have determined this athlete has sustained a contusion to the lower right quadrant. What actions would you take at this time? (Please select and prioritize your choices.)

__ 12. Apply an ice pack to the injured area.

__ 13. Apply a compression wrap to the injured area.

__ 14. Massage the athlete's lumbar area.

__ 15. Massage the athlete's abdominal area.

__ 16. Assist the athlete to walk off the field if he is able to do so.

__ 17. Apply a neoprene rib belt.

__ 18. Position the athlete in supine with his knees bent.

__ 19. Monitor the athlete for any changes in pain intensity.

__ 20. Take the athlete's pulse and blood pressure.

Section C

You follow up with the athlete the next day in the training room. He states he is sore, but has less pain today. How would you treat this athlete at this time? (Please select and prioritize your choices.)

__ 21. Continue to apply ice to the injured area.

__ 22. Begin to apply moist heat packs.

__ 23. Manually muscle test the abdominal muscles.

__ 24. Re-evaluate the injury.

__ 25. Have the athlete drink a glass of Gatorade.

__ 26. Pad the area for activity.

__ 27. Have the athlete begin exercises on an upper body ergometer.

PROBLEM XIX

Opening Scene

You are covering a high school field hockey game when one of your players gets hit hard in the mouth with a stick. She comes running off the field with her hand covering her mouth. There is a copious amount of blood on her face and hands.

Section A

What steps would you take during your initial evaluation of this athlete? (Please select and prioritize your choices.)

__ 1. Rinse the athlete's mouth out with water.

__ 2. Clean the athlete's mouth out with a paper towel.

__ 3. Don latex gloves.

__ 4. Ask the athlete why she is crying.

__ 5. Ask the athlete if she was wearing a mouthguard.

__ 6. Review the school's liability insurance.

__ 7. Observe the mouth, lips, and surrounding structures for lacerations or abrasions.

__ 8. Palpate the mouth and surrounding structures for deformity.

__ 9. Ask a student trainer to get a cervical collar.

__ 10. Have the athlete open and close her mouth.

Section B

During your initial evaluation, you observe the athlete is missing a front tooth. One of the athlete's teammates comes to the sidelines with the tooth in her hand. What actions would you take at this time? (Please select and prioritize your choices.)

__ 11. Ask the officials to stop the game.

__ 12. Have a student trainer take the athlete to the school nurse.

__ 13. Discuss your findings with the athlete's parents.

__ 14. Call your team physician for guidance.

__ 15. Apply an ice pack to the mouth area.

__ 16. Apply a cotton plug between the lip and injured gum.

__ 17. Place the tooth in a container of sterile saline solution.

__ 18. Rinse the tooth off with water.

__ 19. Send the athlete with the tooth to a dentist in less than 30 minutes.

__ 20. Discard the tooth.

__ 21. Place the athlete in a sidelying position.

PROBLEM XX

Opening Scene

A wrestler comes to the training room during his off-season and asks you to help him lose 15 pounds. This athlete had attempted to lose a significant amount of weight before and failed.

Section A

How would you advise the wrestler in his initial steps to lose the weight safely? (Please select and prioritize your choices.)

__ 1. Have the athlete consume a protein diet once a day in addition to his regular diet.

__ 2. Measure the athlete's percent body fat using calipers.

__ 3. Have the athlete read the *American Heart Association Cookbook*.

__ 4. Send the athlete to an acupuncturist.

__ 5. Have the athlete keep a log of what he eats on a daily basis.

__ 6. Monitor the athlete's weight loss progress once a week.

__ 7. Put the athlete on a fasting diet for 2 days.

__ 8. Make sure the athlete drinks eight glasses of water daily.

__ 9. Weigh the athlete prior to beginning his program.

__ 10. Have the athlete sit in a sauna.

__ 11. Monitor the athlete's exercise program.

__ 12. Assist the athlete in developing a balanced diet.

__ 13. Have the athlete wear a rubber suit while running.

__ 14. Put the athlete on a lower extremity strengthening program.

Section B

The athlete successfully loses the weight. How would you go about advising the athlete in maintaining his current weight? (Please select and prioritize your choices.)

___ 15. Continue to monitor the athlete's food intake via a log.

___ 16. Have the coach monitor the athlete's food intake.

___ 17. Have the athlete drink eight glasses of water a day.

___ 18. Have the athlete double his exercise session in duration.

___ 19. Have the athlete take laxatives.

___ 20. Refer the athlete to a sports nutritionist.

___ 21. Encourage the athlete to eat four to six small balanced meals a day.

___ 22. Put the athlete on an upper body strength program.

Chapter V

PRACTICAL PRACTICE SAMPLE QUESTIONS

You will need two partners and a stopwatch or wristwatch to practice for this section of the exam. One partner will play the role of the model, and the other partner will be the examiner. Have the partner who is playing the examiner read through a few of the questions to him- or herself first and collect any necessary items to complete the tasks on which you intend to work. For example, if you are required to tape a knee, you will need the appropriate selection of supplies. Try to avoid having your partners "help" you by giving you hints, either verbally or non-verbally, along the way. The idea is for you to become confident in your skills and speed of execution. Go over any mistakes you have made after you have totally completed this practice section.

Each task will be assigned a specific time limitation. You must correctly perform 90% of the steps to pass each task, except for Problems X and XIV, which must be correctly demonstrated in full.

PRACTICAL SAMPLE QUESTIONS

Problem I

A soccer player mildly strains his right hip flexor during a game. The athlete needs his leg wrapped in an elastic bandage to make him more comfortable prior to returning to play. You have 2 minutes to perform this task.

   A. Is the athlete positioned in standing with the involved leg slightly flexed and internally rotated?

   Yes ___ No ___

   B. Was a 6 inch elastic wrap selected?

   Yes ___ No ___

   C. Was the elastic wrap started at the upper part of the inner thigh and brought around to the posterior aspect of the thigh?

   Yes ___ No___

   D. Was the wrap anchored onto the opposite iliac crest?

   Yes ___ No ___

   E. Does the wrap prevent excessive hip extension?

   Yes ___ No ___

Passing score = 4 correct answers

Problem II

An athlete comes to the athletic training room after undergoing an arthroplasty of his left shoulder. Using a goniometer, measure the range of motion of shoulder flexion (normal active range of motion is 0° to 180°). Please report your measurement to the examiner. (Note: The examiner should take the initial reading.) You have 2 minutes to perform this task.

   A. Is the athlete positioned in supine?

        Yes ___ No ___

   B. Is the axis of the goniometer aligned through the humeral head?

        Yes ___ No ___

   C. Is the stationary arm of the goniometer aligned parallel to the trunk?

        Yes ___ No ___

   D. Is the movable arm aligned parallel to the humeral shaft siting the lateral epicondyle?

        Yes ___ No ___

   E. Is the trainer's recording within 5° of the examiner's reading?

        Yes ___ No ___

Passing score = 4 correct answers

Problem III

This next task is to test your palpation skills. With a skin-marker or small pieces of athletic tape, place a mark on the following anatomical landmarks of the lower extremity. You have 2 minutes to perform this task.

   A. The anterior talofibular ligament.

        (Correct?) Yes ___ No ___

   B.   Gerdy's tubercle.

        (Correct?) Yes ___ No ___

   C. The anterior superior iliac spine.

        (Correct?) Yes ___ No ___

   D. The popliteal fossa.

        (Correct?) Yes ___ No ___

   E. The quadriceps tendon.

        (Correct?) Yes ___ No ___

   F.   The lateral collateral ligament of the knee.

        (Correct?) Yes ___ No ___

   G. The medial malleolus.

        (Correct?) Yes ___ No ___

   H. The deltoid ligament of the ankle.

        (Correct?) Yes ___ No ___

   I.   The greater trochanter of the femur.

        (Correct?) Yes ___ No ___

   J.   The medial border of the patella.

        (Correct?) Yes ___ No ___

   K. The lateral head of the gastrocnemius.

        (Correct?) Yes ___ No ___

L. The first ray of the foot.

(Correct?) Yes ___ No ___

M. The navicular of the foot.

(Correct?) Yes ___ No ___

N. The base of the fifth metatarsal.

(Correct?) Yes ___ No ___

O. The tendon of the biceps femoris.

(Correct?) Yes ___ No ___

P. The fibular head.

(Correct?) Yes ___ No ___

Passing score = 14 correct answers

Problem IV

A gymnast reports to the athletic training room after sustaining a knee injury during practice. To test the integrity of the medial collateral ligament, you must perform a valgus stress test. Demonstrate this test just as you would on an injured athlete. You have 3 minutes to perform this test.

A. Is the athlete positioned in supine?

Yes ___ No ___

B. Is the involved leg extended?

Yes ___ No ___

C. Has the trainer stabilized the distal limb with one hand?

Yes ___ No ___

D. Has the trainer placed his or her other hand over the lateral joint line?

Yes ___ No ___

E. Has the trainer applied adequate force in the appropriate direction with the knee in full extension?

Yes ___ No ___

F. Has the trainer applied adequate force in the appropriate direction at 30° of flexion?

Yes ___ No ___

Passing score = 5 correct answers

Problem V

A basketball player has been participating in a rehabilitation program for a hamstring strain. Prior to allowing the player to return to playing, the athletic trainer should test the strength of the hamstrings to be sure they are of equal strength to the uninvolved side and are pain free to resistance. Demonstrate a manual muscle test for the hamstrings just as you would on an athlete. You have 2 minutes to perform this task.

A. Is the athlete positioned in prone?

Yes ___ No ___

B. Did the trainer have the athlete first move the limb actively from full knee extension to full knee flexion?

Yes ___ No ___

C. Has the trainer stabilized the posterior thigh with one hand?

Yes ___ No ___

D. Has the trainer placed his or her hand on the posterior aspect of the distal lower leg?

Yes ___ No ___

E. Was the proper force applied to resist knee flexion (in neutral)?

Yes ___ No ___

F. Did the trainer position the lower leg in internal rotation to resist the medial hamstrings?

Yes ___ No ___

G. Did the trainer position the lower leg in external rotation to resist the lateral hamstrings?

Yes ___ No ___

Passing score = 6 correct answers

Problem VI

This task will require you to properly fit a football helmet on a player. Proceed through all the steps, verbalizing each step to the examiner until the fitting process is complete. Inform the examiner when you are done. You have 3 minutes to perform this task.

A. Did the trainer verbalize he or she would wet the player's hair to simulate playing conditions and ensure a proper fit?

Yes ___ No ___

B. Did the trainer apply the helmet from the back to the front and check to make sure the helmet fits snugly with no gaps between the pads and the head or face?

Yes ___ No ___

C. Did the trainer check to see if the helmet covers the base of the skull?

Yes ___ No ___

D. With the chin strap in place, did the trainer pull down on the face mask to make sure the helmet does not move?

Yes ___ No ___

E. Did the trainer push down on the helmet to make sure there is no movement?

Yes ___ No ___

F. Did the trainer attempt to rock the helmet back and forth to check for any movement?

Yes ___ No ___

G. Did the trainer attempt to rotate the helmet to check for any movement?

Yes ___ No ___

H. Did the trainer check to see if the front edge of the helmet is no less than two finger widths above the eyebrows?

Yes ___ No ___

I. Did the trainer check to see if the jaw pads fit snugly against the face?

Yes ___ No ___

J. Did the trainer check to see if the face mask is three finger widths from the nose?

Yes ___ No ___

K. Did the trainer check to see that the ear holes are aligned?

Yes ___ No ___

L. Did the trainer check to make sure the chin straps were properly adjusted?

Yes ___ No ___

Passing score = 11 correct answers

Problem VII

A lacrosse player is recovering from Achilles' tendinitis of the right lower leg. This athlete will need to be taped to prevent aggravating the area during play. Demonstrate the proper technique to tape the Achilles' tendon. You will have 3 minutes to perform this task.

    A. Is the athlete positioned in prone with the feet hanging over the edge of the table?

        Yes ___ No ___

    B. Did the trainer verbalize that tape adherent would be applied to the lower leg (after shaving it if necessary)?

        Yes ___ No ___

    C. Has the trainer applied underwrap to the lower third of the calf area?

        Yes ___ No ___

    D. Has the trainer applied anchor strips one third of the way up the calf and around the ball of the foot?

        Yes ___ No ___

    E. Has the trainer applied a 3 inch-elastic strip from the ball of the foot to the anchor strip on the calf?

        Yes ___ No ___

    F. Has the trainer applied a second 3 inch-elastic strip on top of the first, splitting it down the middle lengthwise and wrapping the two pieces anteriorly around the leg?

        Yes ___ No ___

    G. Did the trainer close the tape job with elastic strips around the calf and the ball of the foot?

        Yes ___ No ___

    H. Does the tape job adequately prevent excessive dorsiflexion of the foot?

        Yes ___ No ___

Passing score = 7 correct answers

Problem VIII

A football player has injured his ankle during a game. After having the ankle wrapped for support, crutches are issued. Demonstrate how to properly fit and walk with crutches in nonweight-bearing. You have 3 minutes to perform this task.

    A. Are the tips of the crutches approximately 6 inches from the lateral aspect of the shoe and approximately 2 inches in front of the toe during fitting?

        Yes ___ No ___

    B. Are the crutch handles in a position so the elbows are bent to approximately 30°?

        Yes ___ No ___

    C. Are the tops of the crutches approximately two finger-widths from the top of the axilla?

        Yes ___ No ___

    D. Did the trainer review a tripod gait in which both crutches are moved forward approximately 12 inches and the athlete swings through the stationary crutches with the affected foot elevated?

        Yes ___ No ___

Passing score = 3 correct answers

Problem IX

A football player comes to the sidelines after making a tackle. He is complaining of some neck discomfort and tingling sensations down his left arm. As part of the athletic trainer's initial assessment, an upper quarter screen is performed. Please demonstrate how to assess the motor function of the upper quarter and verbalize each level as it is evaluated. You have 2 minutes to perform this task.

    A. C3-4 Does the trainer resist shoulder shrugs?

        Yes ___ No ___

    B. C4-5 Does the trainer resist shoulder abduction?

        Yes ___ No ___

    C. C5-6 Does the trainer resist elbow flexion and wrist extension?

        Yes ___ No ___

    D. C6-7 Does the trainer resist elbow extension and wrist flexion?

        Yes ___ No ___

    E. C8-T1 Does the trainer resist finger adduction and grip strength?

        Yes ___ No ___

Passing score = 4 correct answers

Problem X

A baseball player comes into the training room following a practice complaining he feels like his shoulder clicks and occasionally feels like it is slipping when he throws hard. To test the integrity of the glenohumeral joint, the trainer performs an apprehension test. Demonstrate this test just as you would on an injured athlete. You have 2 minutes to perform this task.

    A. Has the trainer placed the athlete in sitting or supine?

        Yes ___ No ___

    B. Did the trainer position the shoulder in 90° of abduction with the elbow flexed to 90°?

        Yes ___ No ___

    C. Did the trainer gently externally rotate the shoulder until the athlete demonstrates apprehension (facial grimace or the athlete requests the trainer to stop the motion)?

        Yes ___ No ___

Passing score = 3 correct answers

Problem XI

A gymnast has a subacute left biceps strain. This athlete will need to be taped before participating in her next meet. Demonstrate the proper technique to tape the elbow to prevent hyperextension. You will have 3 minutes to perform this task.

    A. Did the trainer verbalize that tape adherent would be applied to the elbow area?

        Yes ___ No ___

    B. Has the trainer positioned the athlete with the elbow in 90° of flexion?

        Yes ___ No ___

    C. Has the trainer applied underwrap to the affected area?

        Yes ___ No ___

    D. Has the trainer placed anchor strips with elastic tape at the mid-upper arm and mid-forearm areas?

        Yes ___ No ___

  E. Did the trainer apply a checkrein made out of fanned 1.5 inch white tape or 2 inch or 3 inch elastic tape vertically down the anterior portion of the arm?

    Yes ___ No ___

  F. Did the trainer apply additional anchor strips above and below the checkrein to secure it?

    Yes ___ No ___

  G. Did the trainer apply a final wrap with elastic tape to close the tape job?

    Yes ___ No ___

  Passing score = 6 correct answers

Problem XII

A field hockey player comes into the training room with a large abrasion (4 inch x 4 inch) on the lateral side of her thigh. Demonstrate the proper procedure to care for this wound. You will have 3 minutes to perform this task.

  A. Did the trainer verbalize or demonstrate good hand washing techniques?

    Yes ___ No ___

  B. Did the trainer don protective gloves?

    Yes ___ No ___

  C. Has the trainer cleansed the wound thoroughly with soap and water or hydrogen peroxide?

    Yes ___ No ___

  D. Has the trainer applied an antiseptic such as Betadine to the wound?

    Yes ___ No ___

  E. If medication is applied, has the trainer placed the ointment or cream on the pad or dressing (ie, not directly to the wound)?

    Yes ___ No ___

  F. Has the trainer secured the dressing in place with an elastic wrap or tape?

    Yes ___ No ___

  G. Did the trainer verbalize that the contaminated gloves would be disposed of in a biohazard bag?

    Yes ____ No ___

  Passing score = 6 correct answers

Problem XIII

A volleyball player limps into the training room after twisting her ankle on the court during a practice drill. An inversion sprain is suspected. To test the integrity of the ankle joint, an anterior drawer test is performed. Please demonstrate this test just as you would on an injured athlete. You have 2 minutes to perform this task.

  A. Is the athlete positioned in supine or sitting on the edge of a treatment table with the feet relaxed and hanging freely over the edge of the table?

    Yes ___ No ___

  B. Has the trainer stabilized the lower tibia with one hand?

    Yes ___ No ___

  C. Did the trainer grasp the calcaneus with the other hand?

    Yes ___ No ___

  D. Did the trainer attempt to move the calcaneus anteriorly with adequate force?

    Yes ___ No ___

  E. Did the trainer verbalize that a clunking feeling at the endpoint of the movement is a positive finding?

    Yes ___ No ___

  Passing score = 4 correct answers

Problem XIV

A baseball player reports having pain along the ball of his right foot while walking and running. It has now progressed to the point where he is limping slightly. To decrease his pain while he is being treated for the inflammation, a metatarsal pad is applied for use during activity. Please demonstrate the proper technique to apply a metatarsal pad to this athlete's foot. You have 2 minutes to perform this task.

A. Is the athlete positioned in supine or sitting with the plantar surface of the affected foot turned upward?

Yes ___ No ___

B. Has the trainer placed a 2 to 2.5 inch oval approximately 0.125 to 0.25 inch thick felt metatarsal pad just behind the metatarsal heads?

Yes ___ No ___

C. Did the trainer secure the pad with loosely applied elastic tape?

Yes ___ No ___

Passing score = 3 correct answers

Problem XV

During a poorly executed dismount, a gymnast lands on his shoulder. After an initial assessment of the injury, the trainer suspects a potentially serious shoulder injury. To make the athlete more comfortable and for protection, the trainer applies a cloth triangular bandage as a cervical arm sling. Please demonstrate how a cervical arm sling is properly applied. You will have 2 minutes to perform this task.

A. Is the athlete positioned in standing with his/her arm in approximately 70° of elbow flexion?

Yes ___ No ___

B. Has the trainer positioned the triangular bandage under the injured arm so that the apex is facing the elbow joint?

Yes ___ No ___

C. Has the trainer brought the superior corner up over the shoulder of the injured arm?

Yes ___ No ___

D. Has the trainer brought the inferior corner up over the shoulder of the uninjured side, tying it in knot to the opposite corner behind the neck?

Yes ___ No ___

E. Has the trainer brought the apex of the triangle forward and secured it with a safety pin?

Yes ___ No ___

Passing score = 4 correct answers

Problem XVI

A baseball player mildly sprains his left ankle during a game. Following treatment, he is able to return to the next scheduled game but requires his ankle to be taped prior to playing. Please demonstrate the proper technique to tape an ankle to prevent a second inversion sprain. You will have 3 minutes to perform this task.

A. Is the athlete's foot and ankle positioned in maximal dorsiflexion and eversion?

Yes ___ No ___

B. Did the trainer verbalize that he or she would apply tape adherent and underwrap prior to taping?

Yes ___ No ___

C. Has the trainer applied anchor strips around the lower third of the calf at the musculotendinous junction of the gastrocnemius?

Yes ___ No ___

D. Has the trainer applied anchor strips around the foot over the base of the fifth metatarsal?

Yes ___ No ___

E. Has the trainer applied stirrup strips?

Yes ___ No ___

F. Has the trainer applied horizontal strips continually up the leg in either a basket weave form or as continual support?

Yes ___ No ___

G. Has the trainer applied heel locks (with or without a figure-eight strip) for additional support?

Yes ___ No ___

H. Upon inspecting the tape job, are there any gaps visible?

Yes ___ No ___

I. Does the model feel the tape prevents active inversion of the ankle?

Yes ___ No ___

J. Upon removing the tape, are there any noticeable wrinkles that could cause blisters?

Yes ___ No ___

Passing score = 9 correct answers

Problem XVII

Two football players collide on the field while scrambling for a fumble. One player appears dazed as he walks off the field to the sideline. During the athletic trainer's assessment, the cranial nerves are checked. Please demonstrate how each nerve, numbers I through XII, are evaluated. You have 3 minutes to perform this task.

A. CN I—Olfactory. Did the trainer ask the athlete to smell something with his or her eyes closed?

Yes ___ No ___

B. CN II—Optic. Did the trainer ask the athlete if he or she can see his or her fingers in his or her periphery?

Yes ___ No ___

C. CN III—Oculomotor. Did the trainer ask the athlete to track his or her finger up and down and side to side?

Yes ___ No ___

D. CN IV—Trochlear. Did the trainer ask the athlete to track his or her finger up and down and side to side (same test as CN III)?

Yes ___ No ___

E. CN V—Trigeminal. Did the trainer check the sensation of the face (bilaterally)?

Yes ___ No ___

F. CN VI—Abducens. Did the trainer ask the athlete to track his or her finger side to side (similar test as CN III)?

Yes ___ No ___

G. CN VII—Facial. Did the trainer ask the athlete to frown or smile?

Yes ___ No ___

H. CN VIII—Acoustic. Did the trainer check the athlete's hearing (eg, with a watch or a tuning fork)?

Yes ___ No ___

I. CN IX—Glossopharyngeal. Did the trainer ask the athlete to swallow?

Yes ___ No ___

J.   CN X—Vagus. Did the trainer ask the athlete to say "ah"?

Yes ___ No ___

K.   CN XI—Spinal accessory. Did the trainer ask the athlete to shrug his or her shoulders?

Yes ___ No ___

L.   CN XII—Hypoglossal. Did the trainer ask the athlete to stick his or her tongue out?

Yes ___ No ___

Passing score = 11 correct answers

Problem XVIII

An athlete is brought to the training room by his coach and a teammate. His right knee is positioned in slight flexion and a small effusion is noted. To test the integrity of the anterior cruciate ligament, a Lachman's test is performed. Please demonstrate this test as you would on an injured athlete. You have 2 minutes to perform this test.

A.   Is the athlete positioned in supine?

Yes ___ No ___

B.   Is the athlete's knee positioned in 30° or less of flexion?

Yes ___ No ___

C.   Has the trainer stabilized the distal femur with one hand?

Yes ___ No ___

D.   Has the trainer grasped the proximal tibia with the other hand, attempting to move the tibia anteriorly on the femur?

Yes ___ No ___

E.   Has the trainer applied adequate force in the appropriate direction?

Yes ___ No ___

Passing score = 4 correct answers

Problem XIX

An athlete has been undergoing therapy after a significant ankle sprain. Using a goniometer, measure the range of motion of plantar flexion of the ankle (normal active range of motion is 0° to 40°). Please verbalize your measurement to the examiner. The examiner should take the initial reading. You have 2 minutes to complete this task.

A.   Is the athlete positioned in sitting with his or her foot hanging freely?

Yes ___ No ___

B.   Is the axis of the goniometer centered over the lateral malleolus?

Yes ___ No ___

C.   Is the stationary arm of the goniometer aligned with the fibular shaft, siting the fibular head?

Yes ___ No ___

D.   Is the movable arm of the goniometer aligned parallel to the plantar aspect of the calcaneus?

Yes ___ No ___

E.   Is the trainer's recording within 5° of the examiner's reading?

Yes ___ No ___

Passing score = 4 correct answers

Problem XX

This task will require you to properly fit football shoulder pads on a player. Proceed through all the steps, verbalizing each step to the examiner until the fitting process is complete. Inform the examiner when you are done. You will have 3 minutes to perform this task.

A. Did the trainer verbalize he or she would measure the width of the shoulders to determine the proper size of the shoulder pads?

Yes ___ No ___

B. Did the trainer check to make sure that the inside shoulder pad covers the tip of the shoulder and is in line with the lateral aspect of the shoulder?

Yes ___ No ___

C. Did the trainer check to make sure that the epaulets and cups cover the deltoid muscle(s)?

Yes ___ No ___

D. Did the trainer check to make sure that the athlete can raise his or her arms overhead without the pads sliding back and forth?

Yes ___ No ___

E. Did the trainer check the straps located under the arms to make sure the pads are not free to move?

Yes ___ No ___

Passing score = 4 correct answers

Chapter VI

WHAT TO DO IF YOU
DO NOT PASS THE FIRST TIME

There will always be a few candidates who do not pass one section, two sections, or the entire examination. If you find yourself in this position, do not panic. It is important to identify factors that may have led to mistakes.

Although it is understandable to feel sad, frustrated, or angry, it is best not to dwell too long on what cannot be changed and focus your energy on the next examination being offered. The NATABOC certification examination is offered up to five times a year at various sites across the country. You should allow yourself another 3 to 6 months (depending on your employment situation) to prepare and pass the next exam. You may retake the section(s) you failed as many times as you want as long as it is within 1 year of the date of your last attempt at passing the examination. Keep in mind that you will have to send another application and retake all three sections of the examination if you do not retake the failed section(s) within this 1-year period.

It is very important that you submit the re-examination form that comes with your examination scores as soon as you are ready. Your CPR certification must be current and all your academic coursework and athletic training hours must be complete when you send in your application. Do not forget to send the application fee and indicate at which site you desire to take the test so you are properly registered. Be sure you are aware of the application deadline; do not forget to mark your calender!

The NATABOC recommends that if you fail one or more sections of the certification examination that you review your results with your endorsing athletic trainer so that he or she can counsel you regarding taking additional coursework or participating in further fieldwork to help you build your skills. This is a good piece of advice, given your supervising athletic trainer should know you the best and can provide valuable guidance. In addition, a list of references that are used to develop the NATABOC examination can be found on the NATABOC website at http://www.nataboc.org/textbooks.html. These books may help you with your studies for your next attempt.

In addition, if for any reason you feel that you may have a disability or handicap that may have affected your performance during the examination, you may request that the NATABOC modify the certification procedures to accommodate your disability. Make sure that you send your request for this accommodation in writing to the NATABOC well in advance of the application deadline so special arrangements can be made for you.

It might benefit you to take a course on stress management techniques (eg, meditation or visualization) to help you reduce your anxiety while studying. It helps to talk things out with friends, coworkers, or your professors, but they may be limited in their ability to provide you with the tools needed to improve your coping skills. If you are finding you are having significant difficulty dealing with not passing the examination or your anxiety level is not manageable, we suggest you seek professional counseling. In general, try to maintain a positive attitude as you study and get yourself reorganized. Keep in mind that you will have a better idea of how the examination is presented because you have already been through it once.

It is also important to notify your employer (if it is relevant) of the status of your examination results. If you are honest and up front, he or she may be more understanding of your situation. Remember that you may not practice as a certified athletic trainer until you pass the certification examination, and to do so will put both you and your employer in jeopardy of a malpractice suit.

If you are determined and want to be a certified athletic trainer badly enough, you will pass this examination. As mentioned before, give yourself the appropriate time to heal and then pull yourself up by the bootstraps and reorganize your approach. Critically examine your strengths and weaknesses and dig in for the long haul. Remember, the word "quit" is never in a true athletic trainer's vocabulary.

SAMPLE STUDY CALENDAR AND DAILY LOG

Sun	Mon	Tues	Wed	Thurs	Fri	Sat
	1	2	3	4	5	6
7	8	9 Review	10 Written	11 Simulation	12	13
14	15	16	17 Review	18 Practical	19	20
21 Check route to site	22	23	24	25	26 Arrive at hotel	27 Exam day
28	29	30	31			

Figure 1. Sample study calendar.

Hour	Thurs, May 7	Fri, May 8	Sat, May 9
6:00-7:00am			
7:00-8:00am	breakfast	breakfast	breakfast
8:00-9:00am	anatomy (UE)	practice emergency procedures with Tim, Mike, Bob	practice evaluations
9:00-10:00am	anatomy (UE)		shoulder, knee, ankle
10:00-11:00am	ankle/UE taping	practice emergency procedures with Tim, Mike, Bob	shoulder, knee, ankle
11:00-12:00noon	knee taping		shoulder, knee, ankle
12:00-1:00pm	lunch	lunch	lunch
1:00-2:00pm	nutrition	anatomy (LE)	anatomy (back/neck)
2:00-3:00pm	run	anatomy (LE)	anatomy (back/neck)
3:00-4:00pm	kinesiology/biomechanics	health care administration	psychology
4:00-5:00pm	kinesiology/biomechanics	professional responsibility/ development	human physiology
5:00-6:00pm	physics	swim at pool	biking with Sue
6:00-7:00pm	dinner	dinner	dinner
7:00-8:00pm	rehabilitation/ therapeutic exercise	athletic training evaluation	exercise physiology
8:00-9:00pm	rehabilitation/ therapeutic exercise	athletic training evaluation	movie
9:00-10:00pm	rehabilitation/ therapeutic exercise	athletic training evaluation	movie
10:00-11:00pm			

Figure 2. Sample daily log.

ANSWER KEY— WRITTEN EXAMINATION SAMPLE QUESTIONS

ATHLETIC TRAINING DOMAINS

Prevention of Athletic Injury and Illness

1. D) A sphygmomanometer is an instrument used to indirectly determine arterial blood pressure.

2. B) The Q-angle is taken by first drawing an imaginary line from the anterior superior iliac spine down the thigh through the midpoint of the patella. A second line is drawn down the midline of the anterior thigh to the tibial tubercle. The angle created by the intersection of the two lines is then recorded. An angle greater than 20° is abnormal, causing excessive genu valgus. Excessive genu valgus may lead to patellar problems in the athlete.

3. A) To test the gluteus medius in an antigravity position against resistance, the athlete must be in side-lying with the affected limb on top.

4. D) Shortening the stride during running may actually decrease the incidence of an overuse syndrome. Overstriding may result in a hamstring pull or knee pain.

5. A) The average range of motion of the knee is 0° to 135°.

6. C) Numbness or tingling in either or both hands in cold weather is symptomatic of Reynaud's syndrome, which is bilateral episodic spasms of the digital blood vessels. The cause is usually idiopathic.

7. D) True leg length discrepancy is measured between the anterior superior iliac spine to the medial malleolus of the ankle.

8. C) To test the hip flexor musculature, the athlete should be sitting. The athletic trainer then applies a force down onto the anterior aspect of the thigh as the athlete resists the movement.

9. B) To test the deltoids, the athlete's shoulder should be positioned to 90°.

10. C) Scoliosis is a lateral curvature of the spine with rotation of the vertebrae around its long axis. The ribs may become prominent on the convex side of the curve (rib hump) as the vertebral bodies rotate toward the convex side and the spinous processes rotates toward the concave side of the curve.

11. C) If there is an injury to the long thoracic nerve, which innervates the serratus anterior muscle, the scapula cannot be protracted and it will result in winging, which is a prominence of the vertebral border of the scapula.

12. C) Bracing for structural scoliosis may be effective up to approximately age 18. After this age, the epiphyseal plates close and external devices for correction do not work well.

13. C) An arm span that is greater than the individual's height, pectus carinatum or excavatum, a high-arched palate, significant height, and myopia are all signs of Marfan's syndrome.

14. C) Vital capacity is defined as the maximum amount of air that can be expired after a maximum inspiration.

15. D) Myopia is nearsightedness.

16. D) The liver detoxifies the blood of metabolic byproducts, participates in the metabolism of carbohydrates, and produces albumin, clotting factors and plasma transport proteins.

17. B) The average range of VO_2 max for the average collage athlete is 45 to 60 mL/kg/min.

18. D) Measuring the heart rate during submaximal stress testing is used to indirectly determine the VO_2 max. It is known that heart rate rises linearly with increasing workloads.

19. D) The oxygen consumed by the athlete during the recovery phase of exercise replenishes the oxygen levels in the tissue fluids, increases the myoglobin in the muscles to re-activity levels, and restores the venous oxyhemoglobin to pre-exercise levels.

20. D) Measuring the maximal O_2 consumption during exercise is a good way to determine the athlete's ability to adapt to increased metabolic demands. Adequate pulmonary diffusion, appropriate vascular adaptation, and good physical condition of the active musculature all contribute to the athlete's ability to maintain homeostasis during exercise.

21. D) The Harvard step test, progressive pulse rate test, and the Cooper 12-minute run-walk test are all classified as submaximal stress tests.

22. D) Skin-fold measurements for estimating body fat are routinely taken from the biceps and triceps areas, and the suprailiac and subscapular areas.

23. D) The ability to dissipate heat by evaporation is severely limited in a hot, humid environment because evaporation cannot occur unless volumes of dry air are available to absorb the water vapor given off.

24. D) Running short distances stimulates the breakdown of phosphocreatinine into phosphorus and creatinine in the muscle and glycogen and glucose to breakdown into lactic acid, allowing for the muscles to work for short durations of time.

25. C) Power equals force times distance. It is the intensity at which a muscle is able to perform work.

26. C) As a result of prolonged training and conditioning, the heart may increase in size to meet the increased demands.

27. B) The formula for calculating target heart rate is: 220 – 25 (athlete's age) = 195 x 80% = 156 BPM.

28. D) It takes between 15 to 30 minutes of a warm-up period to prepare the body for athletic competition. This warm-up period varies with each athlete and may have to be extended with an older athlete.

29. D) The average amount of calories an athlete expends in a day is between 2200 and 4400 calories.

30. A) These percentages are according to USDA guidelines.

31. D) Because specific types of food and timing of the pre-event meal are significant to performance, it is important the athletic trainer, coach, and athlete are all involved in its proper planning.

32. B) It takes a minimum of 3 to 4 hours for food to digest. Fats take as long as 5 hours to leave the stomach. Proteins take as long as 3 hours and carbohydrates take approximately 2 hours to pass into the upper small intestine.

33. C) It is crucial that an athlete stay properly hydrated to maintain homeostasis and proper cardiac function. Average water needs for an adult is approximately 1 mL/Kcal burned. This equals approximately 2.4 liters for a 2400 Kcal energy output. Since the body does not conserve water well, it must be frequently replenished, especially while competing.

34. D) Female athletes who do not menstruate on a regular basis or those who vigorously exercise may eventually sustain severe bone loss, and osteoporosis may result. Calcium supplement of 1500 mg/day may effectively reduce the bone loss in the total skeleton and reduce the need for estrogen therapy.

35. A) The idea behind a carbohydrate-loading program is to increase the storage of glycogen in the muscles to improve performance in the endurance athlete. The athlete should consume a meal that is high in carbohydrates (such as pasta) and only lightly exercise the day before competition.

36. D) The primary adverse side effect of the NSAID group is gastrointestinal discomfort.

37. B) Common side effects of antibiotic therapy are abdominal cramping, diarrhea, nausea, and vomiting.

38. A) Aspirin is administered in 325 mg tablets.

39. B) Side effects of oral contraceptives include nausea and vomiting, fluid retention, amenorrhea, and a feeling of sluggishness.

40. C) A female may develop a condition known as hirsutism, which is the excessive growth of hair in unusual places with the ingestion of testosterone.

41. C) Ultrasound is based on the reverse piezoelectric effect.

42. B) Ultrasound waves cannot be transmitted through air. Ultrasound energy must be transmitted through a coupling medium, such as water or a lotion.

43. B) Convection is a method of heating by which heat is transferred from the source to the recipient by means of movement of the heating medium (eg, air or water).

44. D) The duty cycle is that time in which sound waves are being emitted during one pulse period.

45. A) A moist heat pack is considered a superficial heater.

46. B) Conventional TENS uses a frequency in the 50-100 PPS range with a phase duration of 2-50 μ sec.

47. A) Galvanic burns are the most serious adverse reaction to iontophoresis and are caused by the galvanic current itself.

48. C) The temperature of a paraffin bath should be maintained between 126°F and 130°F to keep it in a molten state.

49. B) Ultrasound converts high-frequency sound energy into heat energy as it penetrates the tissue.

50. D) Ultrasound waves are reflected by bone and absorbed by muscle.

51. B) Inflammation, hemorrhage, infection, and phlebitis are all contraindications for massage.

52. D) Diathermy is used to decreased pain, increase local circulation, and reduce spasms after a musculotendinous injury.

53. A) Scar tissue may be reduced with the use of pulsed ultrasound.

54. B) The inverse square law states that the intensity of radiation from a light source varies inversely to the square of the distance from the source.

55. D) Phonophoresis is the delivery of medication via sound waves and iontophoresis is the delivery of medication via direct electric current.

56. A) The primary indication for cervical traction is to reduce muscle pain and spasm.

57. C) As per universal precautions, the athletic trainer should always use latex gloves when treating a bleeding athlete.

58. A) To avoid the effects of jet lag, athletes should adjust all training, eating, and sleeping schedules to the local time in which they are competing.

59. C) The athletes may play in this type of heat as long as they take at least a 10-minute break every hour and change t-shirts when they are wet to allow for adequate evaporation.

60. C) Otitis externa is a bacterial or fungal infection of the outer ear canal which is characterized by severe ear pain, hearing difficulty, drainage from the ear canal, swelling of the canal, and occasional dizziness. Prevention includes avoiding prolonged exposure to water (eg, swimming/showering) and keeping the ear dry after water activities with acetic acid or a similar drying agent.

61. C) Pediculosis is an infestation of body lice and is usually spread by close sexual contact.

62. D) When fitting an athlete for protective equipment, the athlete's size, skill level, sport position, physical development, and strength should be considered.

63. A) The helmet should not move if tilted, rotated, or turned side to side. The trainer should push down on the crown of the helmet and check to see that the jaw pads and chin strap fit correctly.

64. D) An athlete with renal disease, uncontrolled hypertension, or an acute infection would be disqualified from athletic competition.

65. C) A student athletic trainer must perform any athletic training tasks under the direct supervision of a certified athletic trainer.

66. D) The athletic trainer's daily documentation should include a daily injury log, any treatments administered and how they were implemented, rehabilitation progression, and the athlete's current playing status.

67. D) Only the team physician has the authority to clear an injured athlete so he or she can return to play.

68. C) A tort may be a direct result of an act of omission or commission.

69. B) The coach, equipment manager, and the athletic trainer should all be involved in the selection and maintenance of the athlete's protective equipment.

70. B) NOCSAE stands for the National Operating Committee for Standards in Athletic Equipment.

71. A) The two major categories that football helmets may fall into are the air- or fluid-filled helmet and the padded helmet.

72. A) Maximum protection is provided by a mouthpiece when it is made of a flexible, resilient material and is form-fitted to the teeth and upper jaw.

73. B) The epaulets and cups of properly fitting shoulder pads should cover the deltoids.

74. D) A flak jacket is a piece of protective equipment designed to protect the thoracic area after a rib injury.

75. D) The American Society for Testing and Materials (ASTM) is responsible for setting the standards for eye protection for racquet sports.

76. D) Palm protectors for gymnastics is not considered an NCAA-mandated piece of equipment.

77. B) Only a licensed physician may diagnose an injury and is in charge of overseeing the treatment administered by the athletic trainer.

Recognition, Evaluation, and Immediate Care of Injuries

1. C) The Thompson test involves squeezing the gastrocnemius-soleus complex while the athlete lies prone on a table. The foot should plantar flex when the common muscle belly of these muscles is squeezed. An absence of plantar flexion upon squeezing is a positive test, indicative of a possible Achilles' tendon rupture.

2. B) The radial nerve innervates the extensor carpi radialis longus, extensor carpi radialis brevis, extensor carpi ulnaris, and extensor digitorum of the wrist, which when acting together, extend the wrist.

3. D) The most common type of ankle sprain is an inversion sprain. The primary mechanism of injury is a plantar flexion/inversion movement, which usually affects the anterior talofibular ligament first. As the sprain increases in severity, other ligaments around the ankle become involved (such as the calcaneofibular or tibiofibular ligaments).

4. C) A "burner" is a nerve injury commonly caused when the head is forced to one side while the opposite shoulder is depressed. It usually affects the upper trunk of the brachial plexus. A pinched nerve syndrome may also be caused by a nerve root entrapment, subluxed cervical facets, a bulging intervertebral disc, or a combination of lesions (nerve root entrapment and traction injury).

5. A) A sag sign is positive for a torn posterior cruciate ligament when, as the athlete is lying supine and the knee is flexed to 45°, the tibial plateau sags posteriorly, causing a sulcus just inferior to the inferior border of the patella of the affected leg.

6. A) An athletic trainer's initial evaluation of an injury should begin the moment the injury is witnessed or upon initial contact with the athlete or another individual who might have witnessed the injury.

7. B) The Glasgow Coma Scale is used to determine an individual's level of consciousness or degree of coma. The three indicators of consciousness used are the stimulus needed to elicit eye opening, type of verbal response, and type of motor response.

8. C) The L5 nerve root innervates the extensor hallucis longus muscle.

9. B) A positive Phalen's test is indicative of carpal tunnel syndrome. The athlete is asked to stand with the dorsal aspect of both hands in full contact so both wrists are maximally flexed for 1 minute. Complaints of numbness and tingling in the medial nerve distribution of the fingers is a positive test.

10. C) The Trendelenberg test is used to test for gluteus medius weakness of the hip. The athlete is asked to stand on one leg for approximately 10 seconds and then switch to the other leg. If the pelvis on the unsupported side drops noticeably lower than the pelvis on the supported side, it is a positive finding (ie, weakness of the gluteus medius on the supported side).

11. D) The varus stress test is used to test the integrity of the lateral collateral ligament of the knee. The athlete is asked to lie supine with the knee in full extension. The athletic trainer places his or her hand distally on the lateral ankle and the other hand proximally on the knee medially. With the ankle stabilized, a varus force is applied with the proximal hand. Lateral joint pain and/or increased varus movement with an absent or poor endpoint when compared to the uninvolved side is a positive finding for a torn lateral collateral ligament.

12. B) A positive drop-arm sign is indicative of rotator cuff pathology. The athlete is asked to stand as the athletic trainer passively abducts the athlete's arm to 90° and then instructs the athlete to slowly lower his or her arm to the side. If the athlete has significant pain with the movement or is unable to control the adduction of the arm during testing, the sign is positive.

13. B) The golfer's elbow test is used to identify inflammation in the area of the medial epicondyle. The athlete is asked to flex both the elbow and wrist with the forearm fully supinated. The athlete is then asked to fully extend the elbow. If the athlete complains of pain over the medial epicondyle during testing, the findings are considered to be positive.

14. D) A sign is an objective entity, one that can be measured, felt, seen, smelled, or heard. A symptom, such as dizziness, is subjective in nature. Symptoms can only be experienced by the individual who is affected by the ailment or injury.

15. D) Tactile information alone will not provide the athletic trainer enough information to adequately assess the athlete's functional status. It is crucial that a well-planned, comprehensive evaluation is performed to assess all aspects of the athlete's condition prior to treatment.

16. B) The extensor pollicis longus of the thumb is innervated by the C8 nerve root.

17. D) A positive clunk test is indicative of a possible glenoid labrum tear. The athlete is asked to lie supine. The athletic trainer places his or her proximal hand on the posterior aspect of the involved shoulder and the other hand distally on the humerus. As the athletic trainer passively abducts and externally rotates the subject's arm overhead, an anterior force is applied to the humerus as he or she circumducts the humeral head in the glenoid fossa. A clunking or grinding sensation is a positive finding.

18. D) Recurrent anterior subluxation of the shoulder most frequently occurs with repetitive throwing motions primarily during the cocking and follow-through phases. With constant repetition, the anterior capsule and labrum may stretch or tear, allowing the humeral head to slip anteriorly.

19. B) A pneumothorax occurs when there is the presence of air within the chest cavity in the pleural space but outside the lung. In an intact chest, a pneumothorax can occur if a fractured rib has lacerated a lung or spontaneously if the athlete has a congenitally weakened area on the surface of the lung, which may rupture without antecedent trauma. Sudden chest pain and difficulty breathing as the lung collapses are major signs of a spontaneous pneumothorax.

20. A) The posterior tibial and dorsalis pedis pulses should always be palpated after an acute knee injury to ensure the peripheral circulation of the involved limb is intact.

21. C) An injury to the peroneal nerve of the lower leg will result in foot drop. The common peroneal nerve innervates the peroneus longus muscle, the superficial peroneal nerve innervates the peroneus brevis muscle, and the deep peroneal nerve innervates the peroneus tertius muscle of the lateral aspect of the lower leg and foot.

22. B) A Salter type V epiphyseal fracture is a crush injury to the epiphysis.

23. C) Cranial nerve VII is the facial nerve. It supplies both sensation and motor control to the facial muscles.

24. B) The latissimus dorsi muscle is innervated by the thoracodorsal nerve.

25. D) A second-degree burn is also known as a partial thickness burn and appears as a bright red area with blisters.

26. A) The medial and lateral pectoral nerves innervate the pectoralis major muscle, which flexes, adducts, and internally rotates the upper arm.

27. D) Spondylolysis occurs when there is a defect in the pars interarticularis. A Scotty dog sign is a radiographic finding of spondylolysis. On an oblique view of the lumbosacral spine, there is an outline that looks like a Scottish terrier. The defect in the pars interarticularis appears as the collar on the neck of the Scotty dog.

28. C) The levator palpabrae superioris muscle acts to elevate the eyelid.

29. D) Vision is controlled by the occipital lobe of the brain.

30. D) Jaundice is a symptom of liver disease that causes the skin to appear yellow in color. It occurs when bile cannot be made or excreted normally.

31. A) A Bankart lesion is an injury to the anterior capsule of the shoulder with an associated tear of the glenoid labrum.

32. B) Pronation and supination of the forearm take place in the horizontal plane.

33. A) An aura is a sensation that occurs just prior to a seizure. It may last for a few seconds and appears as a smell, sound, or specific feeling. It acts as a warning to the athlete and generally takes the same form every time it occurs.

34. D) Signs of inflammation include warmth (calor), pain (dolar), redness (rubor), and swelling (tumor).

35. A) Exercise may cause a temporary increase in blood pressure while a change in posture may raise or lower the pressure.

36. B) Type I diabetes is also known as juvenile-onset diabetes or insulin-dependent diabetes, and it usually has its onset prior to age 25. It is not usually associated with obesity.

37. C) Symptoms of mononucleosis include tender lymph nodes, fever, sore throat, and a stiff neck. Low back pain is not a characteristic symptom of this illness.

38. D) Candida is a yeast infection, which causes vaginitis.

39. D) Osteoporosis rarely occurs in an obese individual. Obesity is not considered a risk factor for the disease.

40. C) The normal leukocyte (white blood cell) count is between 4000 and 10,000/cu mm.

41. C) The AIDS virus attacks the T-helper lymphocytes of the body's immune system leaving the individual vulnerable to infection.

42. B) EIA stands for exercise-induced asthma.

43. C) The athlete will hike the hip to allow his or her foot to clear the floor during the swing phase of gait.

44. D) Crutches widen the base of support. This allows for the line of gravity to fall within the base of support, increasing stability.

45. D) Anorexia nervosa is an eating disorder, which is most commonly seen in adolescent females. The athlete consumes a progressively diminishing supply of food until she is malnourished and there is a weight loss of 25% of the original weight. Because of an intense fear of becoming obese, the athlete will not maintain normal body weight for her height and age, even when emaciated. It is a sign of a significant underlying psychological problem.

46. A) There are five emotional phases an athlete may experience after a significant injury or loss. These phases include denial, anger, bargaining, depression, and acceptance. These reactions are normal when faced with a serious injury or illness, and the athletic trainer should allow the athlete a chance to work through each stage without interference.

47. D) Symptoms of overtraining include loss of appetite, decreased concentration, emotional lability, decreased motivation to participate in practices and competition, chronic fatigue, indigestion, and changes in bowel and sleeping patterns. An athlete who experiences staleness should be temporarily removed from activity and allowed time to rest and relax to stimulate renewed interest and motivation to play.

48. D) Signs of depression include insomnia, fatigue, loss of appetite, and a feeling of hopelessness.

49. C) An obsessive-compulsive athlete may perform ritualistic behaviors, such as cleaning his equipment after each game, and repeating specific behaviors obsessively, such as hand washing numerous times after touching a dirty uniform or money.

50. A) An athlete might be prone to injury for a number of reasons, some of which are physical and some of which are psychological. Physical factors include poor strength and endurance, inflexibility, or hypermobility and poor coordination. Emotional factors include depression, family or school problems, or anxiety.

51. A) Dehydration causes a decrease in blood volume, which results in lowered cardiac filling pressure and stroke volume. The heart rate increases to compensate for these adverse effects.

52. B) This meal is high in fat and protein and will take a long time to pass through the digestive tract.

53. A) Consuming a simple sugar prior to an event will stimulate the pancreas to produce high levels of insulin, which in turn will cause a sudden reduction in blood glucose.

54. D) Vitamin C is found in high concentrations in citrus fruits and green vegetables.

55. A) Research has shown that increasing vitamin B6 intake may increase the synthesis of serotonin, thus decreasing the emotional disturbances related to premenstrual syndrome.

56. B) Red meat and pork are the best sources of dietary iron.

57. B) Cola sodas contain caffeine, which is a dehydrating substance. This would not be an appropriate drink when trying to maintain adequate hydration during exercise.

58. A) Vitamin A in large doses consumed over a prolonged period of time may lead to toxic symptoms and death in extreme cases.

59. C) Tetracycline should be taken 2 to 3 hours after meals to avoid the possibility of the drug binding to either iron or calcium.

60. D) The healthy range for percent body fat for the female athlete is between 12% to 14%.

61. A) Water loss of 2% to 3% total body weight will begin to adversely affect athletic performance. Loss of 4% to 5% total body weight or greater are life-threatening percentages.

62. C) Tylenol (acetaminophen) has analgesic and antipyretic properties but is not an anti-inflammatory drug.

63. D) Naproxen is the generic form of the brand name Naprosyn which is a nonsteroidal anti-inflammatory drug. Naproxen does not come in a topical form and is delivered orally.

64. B) Ultram is a centrally acting analgesic drug used to control moderate to severe pain.

65. B) Tinactin is an antifungal medication, which is supplied as an aerosol powder, cream, powder, or solution and is indicated for treatment of tinea pedis (athlete's foot) or tinea cruris (jock itch).

66. D) Aristocort, Kenalog, and Topicort are all corticosteroids that are used to treat the inflammation and pruritic manifestations of psoriasis. Betadine is a topical microbicide agent used for skin and wound infections.

67. C) Butisol is a barbiturate used as a sedative in the treatment of insomnia.

68. B) Xanax is a medication used to treat anxiety and panic disorders.

69. B) Penicillin inhibits the metabolism of bacteria.

70. C) The athlete may feel a burning sensation during an ultrasound treatment if the intensity is set too high, not enough coupling medium is being used, or if the transducer head is moving too slow.

71. A) Acute compartment syndrome is a condition in which soft tissue pressure is increased and the viability of the muscles and nerves of the anterior lower leg are jeopardized. This condition may progress from an initial hematoma usually resulting from a blow to the anterolateral side of the leg to total foot drop as a result of injury to the peroneal nerve.

72. D) It is appropriate during the acute stages of a quadriceps contusion to apply ice to the injured area and put the knee into a slight amount of passive flexion to maintain the flexibility of the quadriceps muscle.

73. C) With deep frostbite there should be rapid rewarming of the body part in warm water between 100° to 110° F. Re-warming of the body part should continue until it is deep red/bluish in color.

74. B) To determine if there is a fracture of the jaw, it is appropriate for the athletic trainer to have the athlete bite down and observe for any malocclusion, ask the athlete to open and close his mouth and observe for movement asymmetry, and palpate the jaw for any deformities.

75. A) An athlete should be immediately referred to a dentist if a tooth has been knocked out, if a tooth has been displaced by 2 mm or more, or when a crown is fractured and the tooth is still alive.

76. A) The liver is located in the upper right quadrant and may be injured with blunt trauma to that area of the abdomen.

77. D) When a male athlete sustains a direct blow to the genitalia, the testicular area may go into spasm. It is best to have the athlete lie supine and flex his knees to his chest until the pain subsides and then apply an ice pack to the scrotal area. Another method of reducing testicular spasms is to position the athlete in sitting and lift him up from behind a few inches off the ground, then drop the athlete to the ground. Once the spasms have diminished, apply an ice pack to the scrotal area. Both protocols are proper.

78. D) When performing two-person CPR, the correct compression to breath ratio is five compressions to one breath (5:1).

79. D) Shock after a severe injury can result from hemorrhage or stagnation of blood.

80. C) A second-degree concussion presents with blurring of vision or unconsciousness lasting from 20 seconds to 5 minutes, complaints of headache with associated amnesia, and the athlete appears confused and often disoriented.

81. C) Cauliflower ear is an injury to the pinna of the ear caused by continuous friction or direct trauma to the auricle, which results in bleeding into the soft tissue of the ear. It is characterized by localized perichondral swelling, discomfort, and deformity of the outer ear.

82. B) An athlete who has a known diagnosis of mononucleosis is vulnerable to a possible spleen injury/rupture if the athlete returns to a sport too soon. The athlete may resume light activity after 3 weeks from the onset of the illness if the spleen is not enlarged or painful, the athlete's liver function studies are normal, no fever is present, and any other complications are resolved.

83. C) If an athlete has increased protein in the urine (most commonly diagnosed by urinalysis during a pre-participation medical exam), it may indicate renal or urinary tract pathology.

84. B) Because stress fractures of the bone can be so small, a typical x-ray will often miss the injury. A bone scan involves injection of a radioactive substance into a vein, which is absorbed by bone. A scanner is used to detect abnormal levels of uptake or hot-spots in the bone, indicating a stress fracture or abnormal lesion.

85. D) A Romberg sign is the inability to balance the body when the eyes are shut and the feet are together. It is a sign of sensory ataxia.

86. D) In this case, it is known the athlete is unconscious from a blow to the head and neck, not from aspirating an object or debris. It is only necessary to perform a finger sweep if the athletic trainer cannot ventilate the athlete and an object that is blocking the passage of air is visible in the mouth.

87. D) The cornea, which is the clear surface covering the front of the eye, is most often injured by a foreign body causing a corneal abrasion.

88. A) The proper position for the fist that is resting on the athlete's body is on the abdomen between the xyphoid process and umbilicus.

89. A) When treating for an impaled object, always leave the object in place and apply a bulky bandage around it to control bleeding and stabilize the object.

90. D) Measuring the amount of motion available at a joint will provide the athletic trainer with no significant information regarding the neurovascular status of the injured limb.

91. B) During a seizure, it is best to keep the area around the athlete clear of objects or spectators and protect the athlete's head and body from further injury. It is important to turn the athlete on his side so if he vomits he will not aspirate. A prolonged seizure is a serious medical situation and it is prudent to call for additional medical support.

92. C) Anaphylactic shock is caused by a severe allergic reaction to a foreign protein or drug. There is a contraction of smooth muscle fibers and increased capillary permeability causing dyspnea, cyanosis, convulsions, unconsciousness and, if untreated, death.

93. C) Brain damage is most likely to occur if the brain is deprived of oxygen for approximately 4 to 6 minutes.

94. A) The carotid pulse is palpated in the groove between the larynx and sternocleidomastoid muscle.

95. C) For compressions to be effective in an average-sized adult during CPR, the sternum must be depressed 1.5 to 2 inches.

96. C) Heat stroke is considered a medical emergency. Heat stroke results in severe hyperthermia with the failure of the thermoregulatory system and dysfunction of the central nervous system. It is a condition that does not spontaneously reverse its course and the athlete may die without immediate medical attention.

97. D) Signs of an acute tension pneumothorax include tracheal deviation, distended neck veins, unilateral absence of breath sounds, and cyanosis.

98. A) Flank pain, hematuria, and difficulty/inability to void are all signs of kidney, bladder, or urethra injury.

99. D) During emergency care of the unconscious athlete, the athletic trainer should make sure the athlete's airway is clear and he or she is breathing normally.

100. D) The most devastating cervical injuries sustained in athletic participation occur from cervical hyperflexion and axial compression.

101. A) The athlete will complain of severe lower right abdominal pain with acute appendicitis and will complain of tenderness to the same area with palpation.

102. D) When transporting an athlete with a suspected spinal cord injury, a spine board should be used to stabilize the athlete during transport and additional medical support should be employed.

103. C) The elbow should be slightly flexed to approximately 30° which places the hand at hip level.

104. C) Endorphins are polypeptides that are produced in the brain and produce analgesia by binding to the opiate receptor sites of pain perception in the body.

105. D) CPR should not be stopped until the athletic trainer is too exhausted to continue, spontaneous breathing and circulation have resumed, or another responsible party continues CPR in place of the athletic trainer.

106. C) Reflex pain experienced in the left shoulder and upper arm after a severe blow to the abdomen resulting in a ruptured spleen is known as Kehr's Sign.

107. A) Although total immobilization of the ribs is not possible, a rib belt or rib taping may help minimize movement and make the athlete more comfortable.

108. C) The classical mechanism of injury for an anterior shoulder dislocation is forceful shoulder abduction with external rotation.

109. C) Athletic taping and bandaging serve many functions including support or immobilization of an injured body part, protect wounds from further injury or infection, control of hemorrhage, and to hold protective equipment in place.

110. C) Continuous taping around a limb may result in compromised circulation.

111. C) The compression to breath ratio during one-person CPR is 15:1.

112. B) Insomnia, shortness of breath with exertion, headache, fatigue, tachycardia, bradycardia, confusion, and edema are all symptoms of acute mountain sickness.

113. A) Applying pressure will minimize the bleeding. Keep the area clean with sterile saline or hydrogen peroxide, apply Steri-strips for temporary closure, and use ice and a compressive dressing to minimize further bleeding. Refer the athlete to the physician for sutures if necessary.

114. D) Placing the tooth in a moist cloth and encouraging immediate implantation is the only means by which to save the tooth. Tooth re-implantation after 24 hours has a poor success rate.

115. C) During an emergency, important information the athletic trainer should provide to the emergency personnel includes the type of emergency, the type of injury that is suspected, the current status of the athlete, the type of care currently being given to the athlete, and the exact location of the emergency (including landmarks).

116. D) With a suspected fracture of the knee joint or of the surrounding area, the splint should stabilize all the lower limb joints and one side of the trunk.

117. A) An athlete may sustain a stress fracture of the bone if he or she is subjected to a few high loads (eg, jumping on a hard floor) or many small loads (eg, jogging long distances).

Rehabilitation of Athletic Injuries

1. C) A manual muscle grade of 2/5 is also known as a poor muscle grade and is defined as completing full range of motion in a gravity eliminated position. A grade of 3/5, or fair, is defined as completion of full range of motion against gravity, and a grade of 1/5 is a trace grade, in which the examiner observes or palpates contractile activity in the muscle, but no movement is present.

2. C) The scouring test is used to test for hip joint pathologies such as arthritis, osteochondral defects, avascular necrosis, and acetabular defects.

3. D) An extension lag exists when the athlete cannot fully extend his or her knee.

4. D) A hand dynamometer is a simple tool used to objectively assess the functional strength of the hand and forearm.

5. A) To test the strength of the piriformis, the athlete should be sitting. The lower leg is resisted as the athlete attempts to externally rotate the hip.

6. B) Average range of motion for elbow flexion is 0° to 135°.

7. B) The biceps femoris is tested with the athlete lying in the prone position. Knee flexion is then resisted with the tibia in full external rotation.

8. A) The S1 nerve root innervates the posterior tibialis, plantaris, peroneus longus, and peroneus brevis muscles, which act to plantar flex the ankle and foot.

9. A) To test the function of the rhomboid major, the athletic trainer should ask the athlete to retract his or her scapula.

10. C) The biceps brachii muscle originates on the supraglenoid tubercle of the scapula (long head) and the apex of the coracoid process (short head). It inserts into the tuberosity of the radius. It functions to supinate the forearm, flex the elbow, and flex the shoulder.

11. A) Hip abduction occurs in the frontal plane.

12. D) The gastrocnemius muscle plantar flexes the foot and flexes the knee.

13. B) The flexor pollicis longus originates on the radius, adjacent interosseous membrane, and coronoid process of the ulna and inserts on the distal phalanx of the thumb. Its primary action is flexion of the thumb.

14. D) Movements of the eyes are controlled by the oculomotor nerve—cranial nerve III.

15. D) The rectus femoris muscle flexes the hip and extends the knee when it contracts.

16. B) The gluteus maximus externally rotates the hip.

17. B) Nerve roots C6, C7, and C8 represent the sensory dermatomes of the hand (from radial to thumb sides respectively).

18. D) The serratus anterior muscle functions to protract the scapula and stabilize it against the rib cage.

19. C) The quadratus lumborum originates on the iliac crest, the lumbar vertebrae, and lumbodorsal fascia and inserts onto the 12th rib and the transverse processes of upper lumbar vertebrae. It functions to laterally flex the trunk.

20. C) The supinator muscle of the forearm is innervated by the radial nerve.

21. B) The extensor digitorum longus extends the toes.

22. B) Food passes from the stomach through the duodenum and mixes with the secretions from the pancreas and liver before continuing on into the jejunum and ileum.

23. C) The median nerve passes though the carpal tunnel at the wrist.

24. C) The ileum is part of the lower small intestine.

25. C) The femoral nerve innervates the pectineus muscle and the obturator innervates the adductor longus, magnus, brevis, and gracilis.

26. B) The abductor digiti minimi abducts the fifth finger.

27. D) The sternocleidomastoid flexes and rotates the head.

28. C) The tibial nerve innervates the gastrocnemius, flexor hallucis longus, and biceps femoris musculature.

29. D) Cranial nerve II is the optic nerve (vision), cranial nerve I is the olfactory nerve (smell), and cranial nerve XII (hypoglossal) is the nerve responsible for movement of the tongue.

30. A) Tissue healing begins with a cellular response, which is associated with vascular changes, followed by phase II, or regeneration of both soft tissue and bone. The third phase is known as remodeling, where there is an increased organization of extracellular matrix and decreased synthetic activity.

31. B) Mast cells and platelets release histamine and serotonin during the reaction phase of an acute injury.

32. C) It may take up to 1 year before soft tissue remodeling is complete.

33. A) The primary location of ATP in skeletal muscle is the sarcomere.

34. C) Golgi tendon organs (GTOs) are sensory receptors found in the muscle tendons that monitor the tension generated in a muscle during contraction.

35. C) During the initial phases following a soft tissue injury, there is transitory vasoconstriction followed by vasodilatation and increased permeability, causing redness and swelling of the area.

36. A) A neurapraxis is the demyelination of the axon sheath of a nerve fiber. This condition will cause a failure of the nerve to conduct impulses, causing a conduction block. It is usually reversible.

37. D) Osteoclasts are cells that resorb bone during growth.

38. A) Cell division for new cartilage growth does not occur in the adult.

39. D) The bone marrow contains immature stem cells that differentiate into red and white blood cells and platelets.

40. D) The athlete will experience the feelings of cold, followed by burning, then aching, and finally numbness.

41. D) A warm whirlpool is a superficial heater. It will only heat the superficial tissues.

42. A) Fibroblasts become active during the regeneration phase of the inflammatory response to begin building collagen.

43. A) Shivering is a method by which the body generates heat.

44. B) External force created by a muscle depends on the angle of the pull of the muscle (ie, when the muscle pulls at right angles to the bone it's moving, the muscular force will be optimal), the length of the muscle (the tension developed with a contraction is greatest if the muscle is at its maximum resting length to start), and the velocity of the muscle shortening (as the speed of shortening increases, the force decreases).

45. D) Proprioception is the awareness of movement, changes of equilibrium, and posture of the body and its segments. The "control center" for proprioceptive awareness in the brain is located in the cerebellum.

46. A) A static stretch requires that the athlete stretch the muscle and hold the position to prevent a muscle injury, which may occur with ballistic stretching.

47. A) The cardiovascular and respiratory systems must work together to meet the oxygen demands of the skeletal musculature during exercise. If the demand is not met by increasing the respiratory rate, the cardiac output must increase to increase the delivery of the red blood cells from the lungs to the heart to the muscles.

48. C) When an athlete is injured, he or she may react strongly to pain and become very fearful of the possibility of being disabled. During this time, the athlete may display signs of overreacting by becoming argumentative or sarcastic. It is important the athletic trainer provides emotional support and allows the athlete to express his or her emotions. It is best to be reassuring and divert the athlete's attention away from the injury.

49. C) Visualization, also known as therapeutic imagery, incorporates the mental rehearsal of a positive rehabilitative experience followed by full recovery. It is a psychological tool used to enhance physical healing after an injury.

50. A) For rehabilitation of an injury to be successful, the athletic trainer must establish a good rapport with the athlete so that the athlete is comfortable and there is a mutual environment of trust.

51. C) An attention-seeking athlete generally will not accept responsibility for him- or herself and enjoys being dependent upon other individuals. As a result, the athlete is demanding and is not satisfied with the amount of time other athletes receive, always wanting more time and attention by the athletic trainer taking care of him or her. This type of athlete is very draining to the health care staff and requires specific boundaries so the staff is not burned out by the athlete.

52. C) Vitamin K contributes to blood clotting because it imparts a calcium binding ability to certain blood proteins such as prothrombin.

53. D) In order to lose 1 to 2 pounds a week, an athlete must reduce his or her daily caloric intake by 500 to 1000 calories a day.

54. C) Cryotherapy is used as an anesthetic and to prevent or decrease the inflammatory process.

55. C) Eddy currents are heat-producing currents that are administered by means of an induction coil or condenser plate of a short-wave diathermy unit. It uses a magnetic field to create these currents within the tissues.

56. D) A monophasic spike waveform delivered in pairs is used with high-voltage pulsed monophasic generators (HVPG).

57. B) Because a moist heat pack is a form of superficial heat, it does not increase the muscle tissue temperature.

58. A) The negative pole or cathode will cause local vasodilatation under the pad, irritation, tissue softening, and edema reduction.

59. B) Inflammation of a body part is an indication for the use of cryotherapy.

60. B) Single-leg hopping would be an appropriate functional skill in assessing the athlete's readiness for play after an ankle injury. Lifting tolerance is not a skill.

61. A) Normal range of motion of a joint must be restored before and concurrently with strengthening exercises during rehabilitation. Limb endurance and proprioception follow in the later phases of treatment.

62. C) Slow-reversal-hold-relax is a PNF stretching technique.

63. D) The hip is moving into a pattern of flexion, adduction, and external rotation during a D1 flexion pattern.

64. A) The proper timing sequence for a D2 extension pattern of the upper extremity is shoulder extension followed by forearm pronation and finger flexion.

65. A) Grade I joint mobilization is appropriate for decreasing pain and spasm.

66. A) An inferior humeral glide is the proper glide to employ when trying to restore or increase shoulder abduction.

67. B) Isokinetic training is generation of a muscular force with observable joint movement that occurs at a constant speed with variable external resistance.

68. D) Cupping, hacking, and pincing are all methods of tapotement.

69. D) Effleurage is a superficial or deep stroking technique used to produce relaxation.

70. C) Proprioception is the awareness of posture, positioning, and movement as the limb is moved through space.

71. D) The quadriceps must contract eccentrically to allow for deceleration of the body in downhill running.

72. D) Post-season conditioning should focus on identifying and emphasizing specific areas of the conditioning components the athlete needs to improve upon.

73. B) During the acute phase of an ankle injury, some form of cryotherapy should be initiated. The water temperature should be set at 55° to 65° F (cold) to prevent swelling.

74. B) The girth measurements of the involved leg do not have to be exactly equal before returning the athlete to full activity, as slight differences are normal.

75. C) Restoration of normal proprioception of the affected limb is the most commonly forgotten component of the rehabilitation program.

76. C) Isometric strengthening exercises are the safest exercises to initiate immediately postoperatively, as there is no joint movement initiated during muscular contraction.

77. B) Jumper's knee is an overuse syndrome of the extensor mechanism of the knee. There is injury to the proximal pole of the patella as it is subjected to the repetitive traction pull of the quadriceps musculature. The quadriceps muscle should be strengthened during rehabilitation to prevent further injury.

78. B) Trochanteric bursitis can be caused or aggravated by a tight tensor fascia latae muscle.

79. D) A tight Achilles' tendon can cause early heel-off or excessive pronation in order to allow the lower leg to move over the foot during running.

80. D) The coach's opinion concerning when the athlete should return to play should not influence the athletic trainer's professional judgment in designing a rehabilitation program and following prudent guidelines for care.

81. A) Range of motion and strength of the shoulder girdle is intimately related to the function of the cervical area.

82. A) The proper sequence for rehabilitating a grade II ankle sprain includes RICE (rest, ice, compression, elevation), stretching exercises, isometric exercises, proprioceptive exercises, and isotonic strengthening exercises.

83. A) Rehabilitation should begin as soon as possible after an injury with the initiation of modalities for pain relief (RICE).

84. A) The first set of 10 repetitions is with a weight that is 50% of the weight that will be lifted in set three when utilizing the Dapre technique of progressive resistive exercise.

85. C) With a diagnosis of patellofemoral pain syndrome, chrondromalacia patella, or subluxing patella, it is important to strengthen the quadriceps with an emphasis on the vastus medialis obliquis muscle (VMO) and the hip adductors in order to improve the tracking of the patella.

86. D) Stretching the anterior chest wall (especially the pectoralis muscles) and strengthening the mid-thoracic musculature (especially the rhomboids and middle trapezius) improve posture and decrease pressure on the structures of the thoracic outlet.

87. A) Williams flexion exercises encourage a position of lumbar flexion, which opens the vertebral foramina, taking the pressure off the nerve root.

88. A) The athlete's body is in a stable, static position while using a recumbent stationary bicycle and does not need to rely on proprioception to perform this activity.

89. C) Scapular musculature should be strengthened first to promote stability before the distal musculature is strengthened to provide mobility.

90. D) Hamstring strengthening should be initiated early in anterior cruciate reconstruction rehabilitation because the hamstrings are the main secondary stabilizers for the anterior cruciate ligament.

91. D) An isotonic knee extension machine is not a closed-chain exercise because the feet are not in contact with any surface.

92. B) Tennis elbow is an overuse syndrome of the wrist extensors. Once the inflammatory process is under control, strengthening the wrist extensors will help prevent a reoccurrence of the problem.

93. B) McKenzie extension exercises are appropriate for treating a lumbar herniated disc, as they encourage the mechanical movement of the disc anteriorly away from the nerve root.

94. B) When performing an abdominal crunch (sit-up), the athlete should cross his arms across his chest, tuck in his chin, bend up his knees, inhale and then exhale as he pulls his torso up toward his knees.

95. C) A rehabilitative brace would be used postoperatively or during rehabilitation after an acute injury.

96. D) Running on a treadmill would most closely relate to the type of activity a soccer player would participate in during his or her sport.

97. A) Mechanical traction is not indicated for treatment of acute sprains and strains.

98. C) The anterior deltoid, triceps, pectoralis major, and latissimus dorsi are all active while performing a bench press.

99. C) The quadriceps and hamstring muscles, the erector spinae and gluteus maximus are all active when performing a full squat with weight.

100. D) The trapezius, pectoralis major, serratus anterior, and triceps musculature are all active when performing a seated military press.

101. B) A grade III joint mobilization is a large amplitude movement throughout the full available range of motion of the joint.

102. A) The SAID principle stands for Specific Adaptation to Imposed Demands.

103. C) A wall is an immovable object and may be used for an isometric exercise. During isotonic exercise, there is a fixed resistance with variable speed of movement.

104. A) Ballistic stretching places high, intermittent demands on the muscle, possibly exceeding its physiological limitations, leading to a muscle tear.

105. C) Plyometric training involves loading a muscle eccentrically prior to performing a powerful concentric contraction. This places the muscle in a fully stretched position just prior to contraction-enhancing explosiveness, which is important in a sport such as volleyball.

106. B) Having the athlete stand on the injured limb on a mini-tramp enhances proprioception by making the athlete react to a slightly unleveled surface. The goal is to have the athlete maintain this position without wobbling or losing his or her balance.

107. D) Because eccentric muscle strengthening requires high muscle tension to be generated, exercising the quadriceps eccentrically is initiated in the later stages of the rehabilitation.

108. A) Full knee extension exercises (from 90° knee flexion to 0° extension) should be avoided in the early stages of anterior cruciate reconstruction rehabilitation because of the high shearing forces placed on the tibia by the contracting quadriceps.

109. C) Partial sit-ups assist in strengthening the abdominals, and trunk extension exercises (with or without resistance) strengthen the erector spinae musculature.

110. B) Any finding that the athletic trainer observes, palpates, or measures is recorded under the objective (O) section of a SOAP note.

Health Care Administration

1. B) The proper referral for an athlete with an eating disorder would be to a psychologist or psychiatrist because of the complex nature of the condition. It should be recognized by the athletic trainer that anorexia nervosa or bulimia is not just a simple nutritional problem but an underlying psychological problem.
2. D) Physical examination forms, permission-to-treat forms, and release forms for athletes with increased risks should be completed and given to the athletic trainer prior to the first team practice.
3. B) A policy is a broad statement of intended action developed by those who are empowered to govern the operation of an organization. A procedure outlines a specific strategy for members of an organization to follow when following a policy.
4. B) The floor of an athletic training room should not be made of wood because of the possibility of it splintering or warping.
5. C) Most schools are not prepared to have a bloodwork station at a pre-participation examination, nor is it necessary or cost-effective for most schools to do so.
6. C) It is prudent for the athletic trainer to maintain some form of documentation on a daily basis.
7. D) An athlete's medical records may not be released to any individual or organization without written permission from the athlete or his or her guardian or parent.
8. C) The athletic trainer is legally responsible for the athlete's health care. The athletic trainer is acting in place of the team physician in making decisions for the athlete's physical health unless there is a situation that is out of the boundaries of the athletic training practice act.
9. B) The athletic trainer should carry professional liability insurance and be familiar with the details of the policy.
10. B) Focus charting is a method of documentation that lists information about an athlete's injury, the actions taken by the athletic trainer, and the response to the athletic trainer's action in a column form instead of a narrative or SOAP note format.
11. D) A physician's letter of agreement is an informal legal contract that outlines the physician's duties and responsibilities. This type of contract should specifically identify the physician as the individual who is ultimately responsible for the athlete's health care.
12. A) Developmental supervision could be considered a "mentoring" approach in which the head athletic trainer facilitates his assistant's professional development while overseeing the day-to-day operations of the athletic training room.
13. D) AIDS is not a bacterial infection.
14. A) An athletic trainer in the nontraditional setting can be considered a manager. A manager functions as an organizer, director, and controller.
15. C) The athletic trainer is ultimately responsible for the care of the athletes in the school under the direction of the school medical inspector.
16. D) The athletic trainer should follow OSHA guidelines in maintaining proper hygiene and sanitation in the athletic training room.
17. C) CARF establishes standards of quality for organizations that provide rehabilitation services.
18. D) A well-written SOAP note should be legible and concise, include many objective measurements, and express progess in terms of functional achievements.
19. B) Documentation such as the athletic trainer's treatment log or SOAP notes could be subpoenaed during a civil litigation suit.
20. D) Capitation is a fixed method of payment made to a provider per member over a specific period of time, regardless of the amount of services provided.

21. C) The most common cause of an indirect sports death is heat stroke (ie, no direct trauma is sustained by the athlete).

22. B) It is the responsibility of the manufacturers or distributors of recreational sports equipment to report any defective or potentially dangerous products to the Consumer Product Safety Commission.

23. A) An HCFA-1500 form is a standard insurance claim form that is accepted by most insurance carriers. It must be filled out thoroughly for quick reimbursement to be obtained.

24. A) It is illegal for an athletic trainer to dispense a prescription drug to an athlete. Only those individuals who are legally licensed to prescribe or dispense prescription drugs may give an athlete a prescribed medication.

25. D) Maintaining accurate records for a high school athlete is the responsibility of the athletic trainer, team physician, and school nurse.

26. A) Tanner's five stages of assessment is an assessment tool to document the maturity of an athlete's secondary sexual characteristics.

27. A) It is crucial that any infected individual, including an infected health care worker, not deny his or her condition and seek the proper medical care when it is appropriate.

28. C) The WOTS-UP analysis (weaknesses, opportunities, threats, and strengths) is a technique that looks at the strengths and weaknesses of an athletic training program.

29. B) In general, a plaintiff has between 1 and 3 years to file a negligence suit. This can vary from state to state.

30. A) A gatekeeper is appointed by an insurance company to oversee the medical care given to an athlete and is usually a primary care physician.

31. A) The UCR (usual, customary, and reasonable) is a charge that represents the maximum amount of money that an insurance company will pay for a service.

32. D) The athletic trainer should carry professional liability insurance in case of a criminal suit.

33. A) Principle I—(1.2) states that "members shall be committed to providing competent care consistent with both the requirements and limitations of their profession."

34. A) The National Safety Council is responsible for drawing sports injuries data from numerous sources.

35. B) The HECC sets standards to certify face masks that are used in ice hockey helmets.

36. C) The three types of state regulations that govern athletic training are certification, licensing, and registration.

37. A) Expendable supplies include items such as adhesive tape, gauze pads, and Band-aids and items that cannot be used again.

38. B) Security, fire safety, and management of emergency injuries must be taken into consideration when developing a risk management plan.

39. C) During the final check-out following a pre-participation examination, the athletic trainer and team physician should review each examination for final approval to participate.

40. C) The individual athlete is the only person who can decide whether or not to participate in a sport according to the Americans with Disabilities Act.

41. D) Bidding is a process where competing vendors quote prices on specific pieces of equipment, and orders by the purchasing institution are usually placed with the lowest bidder.

42. D) It is illegal for an athletic trainer to prescribe and dispense prescription medications.

43. D) A copayment is a percentage of the total amount the policy holder is required to pay for medical services rendered.

44. B) The athletic trainer working in a clinical setting is best suited to treat the physically active patient.

45. C) Any athletic trainer who is in the position to hire a new staff member is governed by federal laws that require all applicants receive equal consideration regardless of race, gender, nationality, or religion.

Professional Development and Responsibility

1. B) Significantly overweight individuals who have large muscle mass are much more susceptible to heat stroke than small-framed, lightweight individuals.

2. C) It is prudent to advise the athlete to place a damp towel between his or her skin and the ice pack to prevent a cryotherapy injury.

3. D) The spread of impetigo can be decreased by having the athlete avoid sharing towels and clothing with other individuals.

4. D) Symptoms of gonorrhea in a male include a tingling sensation in the urethra followed by a greenish-yellow discharge of pus with painful urination. The athlete should be instructed to refrain from all sexual activity until he is treated.

5. C) It is important that the athletic trainer educate the athlete about the treatment process, as it will decrease his anxiety.

6. A) It is proper to have the athlete breathe in deeply at the beginning of the lift and forcefully exhale at the end of the lift.

7. B) Constant pressure on the axilla may cause crutch or "Saturday night" palsy, which is temporary or permanent numbness in the upper extremities and hands.

8. A) Furosemide (Lasix) is a potent diuretic and is banned by the IOC.

9. D) It is wise to suggest to this athlete that he trim his toenails by cutting them straight across. He should do this on a weekly basis.

10. A) When advising an athlete about the proper construction of a running shoe, the athlete should make sure the shoe is made with good quality and that the heel counter is strong and fits well around the foot, the midsole is somewhat soft but does not flatten out easily under pressure, and that the forefoot area has good flexibility.

11. C) It is important to assess the athlete's training schedule and diet to make sure he or she is not overtraining and eating a poor diet. Both may affect an athlete's performance level.

12 C) To prevent re-injury during the rehabilitation of a soft tissue injury, it is important that the athlete not experience pain during active movement.

13. B) Antihistamines have a sedative side effect; therefore, it is advisable that the athlete avoid taking them during the day.

14. D) A well-balanced diet will provide the required vitamins and minerals to keep the athlete healthy.

15. A) Shin guards are a necessary piece of protective equipment to dissipate the force from a direct blow to the anterior leg.

16. B) Wind and wet weather may increase the possibility of hypothermia while exercising in very cold weather conditions.

17. A) Larsen-Johannson disease is an apophysitis at the inferior pole of the patella and is characterized by swelling, pain, and point tenderness at the site. It usually occurs during adolescence. Isotonic exercise is not appropriate for this particular condition, as it may increase the symptoms by causing too much stress on the affected area.

18. D) It is important that the athlete be advised as to when to take his or her medication and which foods/drugs it should not be combined with.

19. C) Cooper's ligaments are the suspensory ligaments of the breast and should be supported during exercise.

20. B) It is appropriate for the athletic trainer to encourage the athlete to express her feelings and needs.

21. C) A fleshy, pink hue of the distal extremity is a normal finding.

22. A) ICER stands for ice, compression, elevation, and rest.

23. D) Heavy strength training work-outs should be limited to off-season and preseason periods.

24. B) Scheuermann's disease is a degeneration of the vertebral epiphyseal endplates, which may cause the intervertebral disc to herniate. An increased kyphotic curve is seen in an athlete with this condition. Extension and postural exercises may help reduce the symptoms of backache in the early phases of the disease.

25. A) It is important to emphasize the importance of good hamstring, hip flexor, and lumbar paraspinal flexibility during the rehabilitation of a lumbar strain to prevent re-injury.

26. D) A potentiating drug is one that is used to increase the effect of another drug.

27. C) Abuse of anabolic steroids will cause a reduction in body fat in the female.

28. B) This behavior violates the NATA Code of Ethics, which, in part, states that "members shall not engage in conduct that constitutes a conflict of interest or that adversely reflects on the profession."

29. A) It is important to maintain good hydration on long flights that cross numerous time zones.

30. B) Athletes should avoid standing near tall objects, such as trees or telephone poles, which may attract a lightning strike.

31. A) Chronic use of chewing tobacco can cause leukoplakia (the development of white patches on the mucous membranes of the mouth and cheek), mouth and throat cancer, bad breath, gum disease, toothbone and enamel loss, cavities, and stained teeth.

32. C) Physical therapists are trained in the rehabilitation of a diverse patient population. The athletic trainer has expertise in the prevention, treatment, and rehabilitation of the athletic and physically active populations.

33. A) Difficulty sleeping, feelings of anger or guilt, self-preoccupation, and constantly feeling tired are all signs of job burnout.

34. D) Providing high quality care to the athlete, publishing articles in professional journals, and organizing professional seminars and conferences are among the best means of educating the general public and other health care workers regarding the role of the athletic trainer.

35. C) The athlete should be advised to concentrate on strengthening his ankles rather than relying on prophylactic taping.

36. A) The most important thing an athletic trainer should do is listen carefully to what the athlete has to say relating to the injury or problem.

37. A) Tinea pedis (athlete's foot) is caused by a fungus infection. The athletic trainer should advise the athlete to keep his feet clean and dry and wear clean socks on a daily basis.

38. B) Pulling the tick off the skin can leave the tick's head still embedded in the skin. Covering the tick's body with mineral oil or nail polish remover will cause the tick to remove its head from the skin.

39. A) An antioxidant is a nutrient that may be found in high amounts in fruits and vegetables and may protect the cells in the body from the detrimental effects of naturally occurring agents such as oxygen.

40. B) It is best to sleep in a sidelying position with the knees bent slightly to avoid pressure on the low back area.

41. C) Hyperextension of the wrist when hitting a backhand shot in tennis is a primary cause of lateral epicondylitis.

42. C) According to the definition developed by the American College of Sports Medicine, sports medicine is a generic term that is multidisciplinary in nature.

43. A) It is wise for the athletic trainer to advise and consult with the team strength and conditioning coach regarding the development of a reconditioning program post-injury.

44. A) Empathy and humor are important qualities that an athletic trainer should possess when counseling an athlete that is in a state of distress.

45. A) The athletic trainer must be competent in classroom teaching methods and should incorporate multimedia and audiovisual aids.

CORE SUBJECT AREAS

Athletic Training Evaluation

1. A) A goniometer is the instrument most commonly used for measuring joint range of motion in the clinical setting. A goniometer may come in a variety of shapes and sizes and may be made of metal or plastic.

2. C) Shin splints refer to a periostitis myositis or tendinitis or a combination of conditions of the athlete's lower leg. They may be classified as anterior or posteromedial shin splints, depending on which group of structures are involved.

3. C) A positive speed's test may suggest bicipital tendinitis. The athlete is asked to stand or sit with the involved shoulder flexed to 90° and the elbow fully extended with the forearm supinated. The athletic trainer should have his or her distal hand on the volar aspect of the forearm and the proximal hand palpating the bicipital groove. As the athletic trainer resists shoulder flexion, it should be noted if there is tenderness or pain over the biceps tendon.

4. B) A physician is the only person who can legally diagnose a medical condition or problem.

5. A) A positive talar tilt test is indicative of a torn calcaneofibular ligament. The athlete is asked to lie on his or her uninvolved side with the involved foot and ankle over the edge of the table and with the knee flexed to 90°. The athletic trainer's proximal hand stabilizes the tibia as the distal hand grasps the talus. As the ankle is initially placed in neutral, the examiner then tilts the talus into an adducted position. If the range of motion in the adducted position of the involved ankle is greater than the uninvolved, the findings are considered positive.

6. D) Whether or not the athlete has medical insurance should not be an immediate concern of the athletic trainer during the history-taking portion of the initial evaluation. Only those pieces of information that assist the athletic trainer in developing a course of action or treatment plan for the athlete should be considered pertinent.

7. C) The L4 nerve root innervates the rectus femoris muscle, the vastus medialis, intermedius, and lateralis muscles, all of which extend the knee.

8. C) A positive Neer test is indicative of shoulder impingement of the supraspinatus tendon or the tendon of the long head of the biceps.

9. A) A positive finding such as a palpable clunk or shift with 20° to 30° of knee flexion is indicative of an anterolateral instability of the knee, secondary to a torn anterior cruciate ligament or torn posterolateral capsule of the knee.

10. B) Spearing occurs when a football player uses the top of his head as a ram, making contact with an opponent. The force is transmitted axially through the cervical spine causing injury. Most cervical spine injuries result from forced hyperflexion, often with a combined rotation movement.

11. D) The most common mechanism of injury for an anterior shoulder dislocation is shoulder abduction and external rotation.

12. D) Glenohumeral instability allows increased movement of the humeral head within the glenoid fossa, which in turn may lead to microscopic damage to the tissues that lie beneath the coracoacromial arch. Resultant edema and microhemorrhage cause a reduction in the joint space and impingement, most commonly of the supraspinatus tendon.

13. C) Plantar fasciitis is an inflammation of the plantar fascia of the foot. It has a variety of possible causes but is commonly due to one or all of the following: pronated feet, poor footwear leading to decreased shock absorption, tight plantar fascia, Achilles' and hamstrings. A metatarsal pad would only be indicated if the athlete also had a diagnosis of metatarsalgia (inflammation in the area of the metatarsal heads).

14. A) Because of the constant purging, the athlete is vulnerable to an electrolyte imbalance and dehydration. Hypokalemia (potassium deficiency) may result from chronic vomiting or laxative/diuretic abuse causing muscle fatigue, weakness, kidney damage, or an arrhythmia.

15. B) Hypoesthesia is dulled sensation to touch.

16. A) Diabetic coma, which results from severely elevated blood sugar levels, results in the athlete feeling drowsy and having an acetone-smelling or fruity breath. The skin may be flushed and dry, the respirations deep, and the thirst intense. This is caused by inadequate insulin intake (ie, insulin-dependent athlete). Although diabetic coma rarely occurs in an active athlete, it can result from a mismanaged insulin schedule, severe infection, or poor diet.

17. C) The McMurray's test is used to test the knee for a tear in the medial or lateral meniscus with the athlete lying in supine. The knee is fully flexed and the tibia is externally rotated with a valgus force and extended, or internally rotated with a varus force and extended. A palpable "click" is indicative of a positive test.

18. A) Impetigo is a skin infection caused by the staphylococcal bacteria. It is prevalent in wrestlers because of their close contact with other athletes. The bacteria can be carried under the nails and in the nose, infecting open skin wounds or abrasions. The lesion looks similar to herpes simplex lesions— a superficial ulcer with a yellow crust. The skin around the lesion appears normal. Treatment consists of local cleaning with soap and water and oral antibiotics.

19. A) Altered vital signs, such as rapid, shallow respirations, ashen skin color, a rapid pulse, and decreased blood pressure are all signs of shock, indicative of a significant internal injury.

20. D) The primary movements of the pectoralis major are shoulder adduction, flexion, and internal rotation. If the pectoralis muscle is torn, the athlete will experience pain and weakness with resistance to these movements as well as pain to palpation of the injured area.

21. D) Signs of pulmonary edema include acute dyspnea, cough, headache, and weakness. These symptoms can occur in athletes who train in high altitudes.

22. D) Most often a pop is associated with an anterior cruciate ligament injury and less frequently a subluxed patella.

23. C) A Colles' fracture is a fracture of the distal radius and tip of the lunate. This usually occurs as a result of a fall on an outstretched arm and hand.

24. B) The Allen test is used to test the integrity of the radial and ulnar arteries of the hand. It is performed by first having the athlete pump his or her hand by repetitively making a fist. The athlete then maintains the fist while the examiner compresses the radial artery with his thumb and the ulnar artery with his or her finger. As the athlete relaxes his or her hand, the radial artery is released, followed by the ulnar artery. If there is a delay in flushing of the radial or ulnar sides of the hand or fingers, there may be an occlusion of the radial or ulnar artery, respectively.

25. B) The lunate is the most frequently dislocated carpal bone, which occurs from a fall on an outstretched hand, which in turn opens the space between the proximal and distal carpal bones and the lunate dislocates to the palmar side of the wrist.

26. A) When the tibia is stabilized in an externally rotated position and a strong valgus force is applied, the medial collateral ligament, medial meniscus, and anterior cruciate ligament are vulnerable to injury.

27. A) Nerve root compression is most appropriately evaluated by electromyography or by a nerve conduction velocity test.

28. B) A papule may be described as a pink/red elevated area on the skin and is solid and well defined. A wart is an infection of the skin caused by the papillomavirus. The lesions are raised flesh-colored or pink papules with a rough surface that tend to grow inward into the foot causing pain while walking.

29. D) The C5 dermatome is located over the area of the middle deltoid.

30. B) In order to expose the anterior deltoid to resistance in an anti-gravity position, the shoulder must be in 90° abduction and in full external rotation. The forearm must be in full supination.

31. D) The most common symptom of lumbar discogenic injury is a sharp, radiating pain down one or both legs. This is caused by a bulging or herniated disc impinging on a nerve root in the lumbar spine.

32. D) An avulsion of the ischial tuberosity will cause local acute pain deep in the proximal thigh/distal buttock area.

33. D) The iliotibial band moves back and forth over the lateral epicondyle of the femur as the knee is flexed and extended. If the iliotibial band is too tight or it overrides and rubs on the lateral epicondyle during downhill running, the bursa between the iliotibial band and epicondyle becomes inflamed. Pain is elicited as the knee is brought into about 30° of flexion. A popping sensation is not a consistent finding with this syndrome.

34. B) The contact phase of the running gait consists of foot strike, midsupport, and take-off. The swing phase includes the follow-through, forward swing, and foot descent. One foot is in contact with the ground during the contact phase, and the leg and foot freely move through the air during the swing phase.

35. B) The tibia internally rotates during midsupport, following pronation of the subtalar joint.

36. B) To check the vascular integrity of the hand after an acute elbow dislocation, it is important to assess the presence and quality of the radial pulse and check for good capillary refill of the nailbeds of the fingers.

37. B) The cardinal symptoms of an extradural hemorrhage include a lucid interval usually lasting for a few minutes up to a couple of hours, followed by a period of lethargy, which may precede a seizure and coma. This is a true medcial emergency and the athlete must receive treatment immediately in order to survive.

38. C) Concussions are classified according to the length of time of unconsciousness and the severity of the signs and symptoms of head trauma.

39. B) Pain with resisted hip adduction and hip flexion with diffuse tenderness and ecchymosis of the medial thigh is indicative of a strain of the groin area.

40. C) With a rupture of the rectus femoris muscle, a large bulge is seen in the upper thigh and there is pain along the entire muscle belly. Extension is limited because of the inability to contract the rest of the quadriceps musculature.

41. C) Burning pain with tenderness to palpation over the lateral epicondyle of the femur is associated with iliotibial band syndrome. If the iliotibial band is too tight, it will rub over this area during running, causing localized inflammation. The Ober test is appropriate for testing for a tight iliotibial band.

42. A) The quadriceps musculature is innervated by the femoral nerve, which originates at the L2, L3, and L4 nerve levels.

43. A) The spinal accessory nerve innervates the upper trapezius muscle. If it is injured, the athlete will not be able to perform a shoulder shrug.

44. A) The pes anserine (sartorius, gracilis, semitendinosus) act together to flex the knee and will weakly internally rotate the tibia.

45. D) Heat exhaustion is characterized by profuse sweating, cool and clammy skin, rapid pulse, a mildly elevated rectal temperature (approximately 102° F), and hyperventilation.

46. C) A complete blood cell count is a test that assesses the red and white blood cell count, hemoglobin and hematocrit levels, and platelet count.

47. D) A -3/5 muscle denotes an incomplete movement against gravity.

48. D) Mallet finger is caused by a blow to the tip of the finger by a thrown ball, which jams the finger and results in an avulsion of the extensor tendon from its insertion.

49. C) Decreased sensation over the dorsum of the foot, inability to dorsiflex the great toe/ankle, and a diminished patellar reflex are suspect of L5 nerve root irritation or injury.

50. A) Active range of motion is used to determine the athlete's willingness to move.

Human Anatomy

1. A) Golfer's elbow and Little League elbow are overuse syndromes of the medial forearm flexor musculature, resulting in medial epicondylitis. This group of muscles originates on the medial epicondyle and crosses the volar aspect of the wrist. Injury occurs with repetitive valgus stresses at the elbow.

2. A) The olecranon process is located on the proximal end of the ulna and extends posteriorly, preventing hyperextension of the elbow.

3. A) The peroneus tertius muscle originates on the lower two thirds of the fibula and inserts on the tuberosity of the fifth metatarsal bone. It assists to dorsiflex the ankle.

4. A) The deltoid muscle of the upper arm is innervated by the axillary nerve.

5. C) The collateral ligaments are most taut in full knee extension and at 30° knee flexion.

6. A) Cranial nerve I is the olfactory nerve.

7. C) The muscles of the rotator cuff include the supraspinatus, infraspinatus, teres minor, and subscapularis.

8. A) The rectus femoris muscle originates on the anterior inferior iliac spine and inserts into the quadriceps tendon, which attaches to the upper border of the patella. The patella is attached to the tibial tuberosity by the patellar tendon. Therefore, the rectus femoris flexes the hip and extends the knee.

9. D) The pes anserinus is described as a goose-foot shaped expansion of the tendons of the sartorius, gracilis, and semitendinosis.

10. A) The subscapularis muscle of the rotator cuff originates in the subscapular fossa and inserts into the lesser tubercle of the humerus.

11. D) The gluteus maximus muscle originates on the upper portion of the ilium, sacrum, and coccyx and inserts on the gluteal tuberosity of the femur and the fascia latae. Its primary actions are to extend and externally rotate the hip.

12. B) The C7 nerve root innervates the triceps muscle, which extends the elbow.

13. A) Cranial nerve VIII, the vestibulocochlear or acoustic nerve, is responsible for hearing and equilibrium.

14. B) Movements of the tongue are controlled by the hypoglossal nerve—cranial nerve XII.

15. A) Continuous pressure on the palm that irritates the deep branch of the ulnar nerve just distal to the canal of Guyon will cause weakness in the muscles of the hand that are innervated by the ulnar nerve.

16. C) The scaphoid bone of the wrist is palpated just distal to the styloid process of the radius.

17. D) The extensor carpi ulnaris is innervated by the radial nerve.

18. D) The hip joint is a diarthrotic or ball and socket joint.

19. B) Knee flexion and extension occur in the sagittal plane around a coronal axis.

20. A) An impacted fracture is a fracture in which one part of the bone telescopes on the other part of the bone.

21. A) A uniaxial diarthrodial joint is a synovial joint that is characterized by hyaline cartilage that covers the articulating surfaces and a synovial membrane that lines the interior of the joint and it moves in one plane only around a single axis.

22. A) The biceps femoris is one of the hamstring muscles and it is active in hip extension.

23. A) Because of the angulation of the articulating surfaces of the facets of the thoracic vertebrae, movement is greatest in lateral flexion.

24. B) The peroneal muscle groups and peroneal nerve and artery comprise the lateral compartment of the lower leg.

25. A) A Baker's cyst is a localized accumulation of fluid in the popliteal fossa of the knee. It may represent a true bursitis or synovial herniation through the posterior capsule.

26. B) The shoulder girdle is comprised of the sternoclavicular, acromioclavicular, glenohumeral, and scapulothoracic joints.

27. A) The coracoclavicular ligaments consist of the trapezoid and conoid ligaments and connect the coracoid process of the scapula to the inferior surface of the clavicle.

28. C) A mortise joint is a joint in which there is a groove or slot into or through which another bone fits or passes (eg, the talus sits between the distal ends of the tibia and fibula).

29. A) The ulnar nerve and artery run through the tunnel of Guyon, which is located in the wrist. It is formed by the volar carpal ligament, the pisohamate ligament (which is an extension of the flexor carpi ulnaris), the hook of the hamate, and the transverse carpal ligament laterally and the pisohamate ligament and pisiform bone medially.

30. A) The muscle most prominently involved with medial epicondylitis is the extensor carpi radialis brevis.

31. D) The multifidi are small muscles located in the back, which extend and rotate the vertebral column.

32. C) The psoas major originates on the transverse processes of the lumbar vertebrae and inserts on the lesser trochanter of the femur. It acts to flex and internally rotate the hip.

33. D) The vastus lateralis originates on the lateral aspect of the femur and inserts into the common tendon of the quadriceps muscle.

34. D) The anatomical snuff-box is located along the dorsoradial aspect of the thumb and is bordered by the extensor pollicis longus, extensor pollicis brevis, and abductor pollicis longus tendons.

35. B) The superior vena cava carries deoxygenated blood from the head and upper body back to the heart.

36. C) Gas exchange of oxygen and carbon dioxide occurs at the alveoli.

37. D) The peroneal artery originates off the posterior tibial artery below the popliteal fossa in the proximal posterior lower leg.

38. C) The odontoid process, or dens, is a projection off the second cervical vertebra, which acts as a pivot point for rotation of the atlas.

39. B) The cuneiform is one of the tarsal bones of the foot.

40. D) The plantar fascia is located on the sole of the foot.

41. A) The origin of the sternocleidomastoid muscle is on the superior/medial portion of the clavicle and the manubrium, and it inserts on the mastoid process.

42. B) The erector spinae is a large muscle comprised of the iliocostalis, longissimus, and the spinalis, which acts as the primary extensor of the trunk.

43. A) The femoral artery, vein, and nerve pass through the femoral triangle.

44. C) The axillary artery is a continuation of the subclavian artery beyond the first rib in the axilla.

45. D) The peroneus brevis assists to plantar flex and pronate the foot.

46. B) The cochlea is an osseous structure of the inner ear.

47. D) The dermatome for the C3, C4 nerve roots is over the superior aspect of the shoulders and posterior neck area.

48. A) The spleen is located in the upper left abdominal quadrant below the diaphragm.

49. A) Little finger abduction is controlled by the abductor digiti minimi, which is innervated by the C8-T1 nerve root.

50. B) The liver and gallbladder are located in the upper right quadrant of the abdomen.

Human Physiology

1. A) The top number of a blood pressure reading is the systolic number, and the bottom number is the diastolic number. The systolic pressure is representative of the blood pressure during ventricular contraction. The diastolic pressure represents the blood pressure during ventricular filling between cardiac contractions.

2. D) The hunting response is a reactive vasodilatation of local blood vessels after initial vasoconstriction This occurs with the application of cryotherapy to a body part.

3. D) Acetylcholine is a chemical found at the endplate of a motor neuron, which plays a significant role in the transmission of nerve impulses at synapses and myoneural junctions.

4. A) The average level of desirable total cholesterol is less than or equal to 200 mg/dL.

5. A) The separation of electrically charged particles causing a transmembrane electrical potential difference is known as the resting membrane potential.

6. A) The two phases of an action potential are known as depolarization and repolarization.

7. B) The primary component of striated muscle is the muscle fiber.

8. C) A motor unit is made up of a motor neuron and the muscle fibers it innervates.

9. A) Type II or "fast twitch" muscle is more prevalent in the sprinter, as this type of activity is more anaerobic in nature.

10. B) Calcium (Ca++) is a mineral that is necessary for proper muscular contraction to occur. Ca++ is a necessary component in the activation of cross-bridging between actin and myosin to shorten the length of the sarcomere in the muscle myofibril.

11. C) During glycolysis, ATP is broken down to release energy. In addition to the release of energy, the byproducts ADP and PO_4 (phosphatase) are released.

12. A) The Krebs cycle is a complex series of chemical reactions in which there is oxidative metabolism of pyruvic acid, carbohydrates, proteins, and fats.

13. A) Sclerotomic pain is a deep, diffuse aching pain, which arises from deep somatic tissues and is transmitted by unmyelinated C fibers.

14. A) Fusiform muscle fibers are arranged in a cord-like shape, while the pennate muscle fibers are arranged in a feather shape.

15. B) Amenorrhea is defined as an absence of flow during menses.

16. A) Laxatives and enemas can lead to dehydration and electrolyte imbalance, which can endanger the athlete's health and impair performance.

17. D) Hemophilia is a disorder in which the plasma coagulation factor VIII is lacking, resulting in abnormal bleeding.

18. D) The rate of passive diffusion of oxygen from the alveoli depends on the partial pressure of oxygen, the thickness of the alveolar capillaries, and the amount of surface area available for diffusion to take place.

19. C) Vital capacity is the maximal amount of air that can be expired after maximal inspiration.

20. A) During the follicular phase of the menstrual cycle, which lasts from day 5 or 6 to day 13, the primary follicles grow; toward the end of this phase just prior to ovulation, one follicle reaches maturity and becomes a graafian follicle.

21. C) The two main phases of menstruation are the follicular or preovulatory phase and the luteal or postovulatory phase.

22. D) The pulp of a tooth is innervated, not the enamel.

23. D) By 4 weeks, a large laceration will heal by secondary healing. Areas of tissue loss are filled with scar tissue.

24. B) The stimulation of the periqueductal gray area (PGA) of the midbrain and raphe nucleus of the pons and medulla during injury will cause analgesia. Endorphins and enkephalins are produced in these two areas of the brain.

25. B) It may take up to 1 year for a ligament to completely heal with scar maturation.

26. C) To avoid hypoglycemia and insulin shock from taking too much insulin and metabolizing significant amounts of glycogen during exercise, the athlete should consume a snack of a complex carbohydrate and protein prior to exercise.

27. A) Cold therapy used in an acute injury will decrease the local metabolic rate.

28. B) If a scaphoid fracture is not properly immobilized, aseptic necrosis may occur and the fracture will not heal.

29. C) Hematuria means "blood in the urine."

30. C) The scalenes are striated muscle and have an arrangement of contractible proteins in a cross-striated pattern.

31. D) The valsalva effect occurs when the athlete holds his or her breath during the contraction, which increases the intrathoracic pressure and causes a dramatic rise in blood pressure.

32. A) Ballistic stretching causes constant stimulation of the muscle spindles, which causes continuous resistance to further stretching. A muscle must be stretched a long enough time to stimulate the Golgi tendon organs.

33. B) The adrenal glands, which are part of the endocrine system, are responsible for secreting the hormones cortisol, epinephrine, aldosterone, estrogen, norepinephrine, and androgen.

34. B) The primary function of the testes is to produce spermatozoa and testosterone.

Exercise Physiology

1. A) The training effect during exercise is reflected by changes in cardiac output. Cardiac output in the trained athlete is a product of an increased stroke volume and a decreased heart rate.

2. A) Three sessions a week is how often (frequency) the athlete should exercise. Forty-five minutes is how long (duration) the exercise should continue, and 80% of VO_2 max is the intensity of exercise.

3. B) Total cholesterol is comprised of low density lipoproteins (LDL), high density lipoproteins (HDL), and very low density lipoproteins (VLDL).

4. B) The sternocleidomastoids and scalenes assist during inspiration by lifting the ribs to allow for the intake of greater volumes of air.

5. C) The hypothalamus stimulates the thyroid gland in very cold environments to generate internal heat.

6. C) Applying a static stretch to the muscle inhibits the muscle spindle and stimulates the inverse myotatic reflex which originates in the Golgi tendon organs, causing relaxation of the muscle.

7. C) An athlete who is hypermobile/hyperflexible may be more susceptible to joint injuries such as sprains and strains.

8. C) Internal training involves alternating intense, continuous periods of work with periods of active recovery. This type of training is very effective when conditioning athletes who participate in sports that involve short bursts of activity and are followed by a period of recovery.

9. A) The off-season period should be a time when the athlete is not training as frequently or as intensely as the in-season period, but he or she should participate in an activity that maintains a level of flexibility, strength, and endurance.

10. C) The principles of overload, consistency, specificity of training, and proper progression must be adhered to in order to obtain optimal training effects.

11. B) Physiological adaptations to resistive exercise include increased ligament and tendon strength, increased mineral content of bone, and improved maximal oxygen intake.

12. A) When the muscle is in a position where there is maximum interaction of the cross-bridges between the actin and myosin myofilaments in a sarcomere, the tension within the muscle will be at its greatest point.

13. D) Heart rate and stroke volume determine the volume of blood that is pumped through the heart during a given period of time.

14. B) Target heart rate can be calculated by the following formula: 0.8 x (220-age), or 0.8 x (220-20) = 160.

15. B) Contract-relax requires that the antagonist muscles contract isotonically just prior to the "relax" (stretch) phase of the exercise.

16. D) The triceps and pectoralis major must contract concentrically during the "lift" phase of a bench press.

17. C) Circuit training is one of the best means of improving muscle strength and flexibility because it includes weight training, flexibility, and calisthenic exercises at various stages.

18. C) The hypothalamus is responsible for thermoregulation of the body.

19. B) Periodization includes the following phases: postseason, off-season, preseason, and in-season conditioning.

20. C) A proper cool down aids the return of blood to the heart and assists in decreasing lactic acid levels in the muscle.

21. A) Plyometric exercises emphasize a quick eccentric stretch prior to a forceful concentric contraction and are useful in building power.

22. C) The amount of testosterone present in the body has a significant impact on the amount of hypertrophy that will occur with weight training.

23. A) The greatest loss of heat from the body occurs at the head and neck. It is wise to keep these areas well-covered in cold weather.

24. D) Those individuals with blonde or light hair and fair complexions are much more susceptible to severe sunburn as a result of prolonged exposure to ultraviolet light. This type of athlete should use a sunscreen that has an SPF of 15 or greater.

25. C) The ozone levels are most diminished in the late afternoon because of the lower temperatures and decreased amount of traffic on the roads.

26. A) An athlete with the sickle-cell trait who trains in high altitudes is susceptible to an enlarged or ruptured spleen.

27. A) Because sweat contains a lower concentration of salt than the blood, there is a much greater loss of water when the athlete sweats. Therefore, fluids, especially water, should be unlimited.

28. C) Plyometric exercises include eccentric exercise, which are the most common cause of DOMS.

29. B) Hilton's law states that the joint capsule, the muscles that move that joint, and the skin that covers that joint are supplied by the same nerve source.

30. D) A protein level of "trace" or +1 by urinalysis is not considered an abnormal finding in an adolescent.

31. A) Women have a lower strength-body weight ratio (due to a higher percent of body fat) than men.

32. D) There is increased mitochondrial density in the skeletal muscle with endurance exercise.

33. B) During a 400 meter sprint, which lasts approximately 45 seconds to 1 minute, the ATP-CP system is the predominant source of energy.

34. C) The diastolic blood pressure should remain close to resting levels during endurance exercises.

35. A) Hemolysis is the destruction of red blood cells caused by the repeated impact of the foot on the ground.

Biomechanics

1. D) A contraction that occurs as the muscle is shortening is known as a concentric contraction. An eccentric muscle occurs as the muscle lengthens against resistance.

2. A) The foot becomes a rigid lever in preparation for push-off during gait when the foot is supinated in midstance.

3. B) The knee has 2° of freedom allowing for flexion and extension in the sagittal plane and rotation in the horizontal plane.

4. B) During shoulder abduction, the humerus and scapula move simultaneously. This is known as scapulohumeral rhythm. For every 30° of shoulder abduction, 20° of motion occurs at the glenohumeral joint and 10° occurs with the scapula rotating on the thorax. During shoulder abduction, the scapula contributes 60° of movement, while the remaining 120° occurs at the glenohumeral joint.

5. B) The agonistic muscle is the primary mover while the antagonistic muscle is the muscle that causes the opposite action (ie, the quadriceps is the agonist muscle and the hamstrings are the antagonistic musculature during knee extension).

6. C) The most common lever system that exists in the body is the third lever system, where the point of attachment of the muscle causing the motion is closer to the joint axis than the resisting motion (ie, biceps flexing the forearm against gravity).

7. D) The movement arm of a force is always greatest when the angle of application is at 90° to the lever being moved.

8. A) An anatomic pulley (such as the patella) can change the direction of the muscle force, but not the magnitude of the force.

9. A) Muscular tension may be increased by increasing the frequency of the motor units firing or by increasing the number of motor units that are simulated.

10. C) Pronation of the foot is a complex movement. It is a combination of eversion, abduction, and dorsiflexion.

11. B) Plantar flexion of the ankle is an example of a second-class lever (ie, the resistance arm is shorter than the force arm).

12. C) Each lever has a force arm, which is the perpendicular distance from the line of force to the axis, and a resistance arm, which is the perpendicular distance from the resistance to the axis.

13. D) Running utilizes linear motion of the entire body and angular motion of the arms and legs.

14. B) Momentum = mass x velocity. Momentum is the force of motion that is acquired by a moving body as a result of its continued motion.

15. D) Potential energy is energy that is stored in a body when it is at rest. The amount of potential energy a body has depends on its position in space. Kinetic energy is the energy of a body in motion.

16. A) Cervical rotation occurs in the horizontal (transverse) plane around a vertical (longitudinal) axis of motion.

17. D) Applying an external force parallel to the tibia will result only in a distraction force.

18. D) An avulsion fracture of a bone is caused when tissue and bone are stretched and tension is produced beyond its yield point. This is known as a stretching injury.

19. A) This situation results in an isometric contraction.

20. B) The carpometacarpal joint is a saddle joint. A saddle joint has one articulating surface that is concave and one articulating surface that is convex.

21. B) The maximum degrees of freedom (number of axes of movement) a joint can have is 3°.

22. C) The elbow joint is a hinge joint, or ginglymus joint, and has 1° of freedom.

23. D) The frontal plane divides the body into anterior and posterior parts.

24. B) When performing a push-up, the distal end of the upper extremity is in a fixed position.

25. A) The tibia externally rotates on the femur during knee extension. This action is known as the screw-home mechanism.

26. A) With compressive loading, the articular surfaces are brought closer together.

27. D) Loading of a joint that is unstable as a result of ligament rupture produces abnormally high stresses on the joint cartilage.

28. C) Shoulder abduction occurs in the frontal plane around an anterior-posterior axis.

29. D) In the anatomic position, hip rotation occurs in the horizontal plane around a vertical axis.

30. B) A spiral fracture occurs when the foot is planted on the ground and the body is violently rotated. The bone breaks in an S-shaped line. The mechanism of injury is a torsion force.

31. B) Blisters may form in the epidermal layer of the skin as a result of continuous friction to the area.

Psychology

1. B) Progressive muscle relaxation is a relaxation technique by which the athlete learns to manage anxiety and control pain. This form of relaxation training incorporates systematically tensing and relaxing muscles in groups (such as the thighs and buttocks). This technique, when practiced routinely, allows the athlete to tune into his or her body reactions and gain more control of these reactions.

2. B) A passive-aggressive personality procrastinates, makes excuses for delays, and tends to criticize individuals he or she is dependent on, but cannot separate from their company. These individuals also lack assertiveness and are indirect with their needs.

3. D) Signs of anabolic steroid abuse include mania and depression, bouts of anxiety and insomnia, changes in libido, and aggressive behavior.

4. B) The general adaptation syndrome is a stress response theory developed by Dr. Hans Selye in which there are three stages an organism may pass through: the alarm stage, resistance stage, and exhaustion stage. The alarm stage consists of the flight or fight response, which prepares the body to take action; the resistance stage is when the body directs the stress to a particular body site (such as an upset stomach); and the exhaustion stage is when the body may become dysfunctional because of chronic stress.

5. D) An athlete who is "burned out" may display a variety of physical and emotional symptoms including negative self-concept and attitudes regarding his sport and teammates, chronic fatigue, headaches, insomnia, and gastrointestinal problems.

6. D) The body passes through three distinct psychophysiological phases in response to an injury: alarm, resistance, and exhaustion. The adrenal glands secrete adrenaline, which stimulates the flight or fight response during the alarm stage.

7. C) It has been shown that an abrupt cessation of exercise can lead to "sudden exercise abstinence syndrome," which is characterized by depression, sleep disorders, arrhythmias, eating disorders, and emotional problems.

8. A) In order for the athlete and athletic trainer to have a good relationship, it is crucial that the athlete trusts the individual who is providing his or her health care.

9. B) Having the athlete draw a mental picture of the healing process can have a positive impact on his or her recovery.

10. A) Two methods of cognitive restructuring are thought stopping and refuting irrational thoughts.

11. D) Obsessive-compulsiveness, mild feelings of denial, providing self-worth, behavior that masks feelings of fear, and taking extreme risks are factors that lead to overcompliant behavior.

12. A) Repeatedly rehearsing various plays in his mind while experiencing pain is a means of diverting his attention away from the pain.

13. C) Anger, loss of appetite, and chronic fatigue are signs of depression.

14. C) The athlete must be cooperative and take responsibility if he or she is to completely rehabilitate an injury.

15. A) "Purging" by self-induced vomiting or self-administered laxatives is a symptom of bulimia.

16. D) If the athlete is anxious, it is best to reassure him and not belittle his fear.

17. B) Staleness is characterized by an apathetic attitude, chronic fatigue, restlessness, and an increase in acute chronic injuries and infections.

18. C) Athletes between the ages of 15 to 24, those sustaining a serious injury with a long rehabilitation process, and those with the prospect of losing their position to a teammate, may become severely depressed.

19. A) Teaching the athlete about his or her injury and the healing process can significantly reduce the athlete's anxiety about rehabilitation.

20. C) This athlete is demonstrating denial of his condition.

21. C) Arranging the rehabilitation sessions around the athlete's daily routine will help the athlete to be more compliant.

22. D) Athletes who have little perceived control over their health care will tend to experience a greater amount of stress than those who feel they have some control over their environment.

23. A) A ritualistic cleaning of equipment is a sign of an obsessive-compulsive disorder.

24. B) Biofeedback is a technique that reflects the athlete's efforts to control a specific physiological response such as muscular tension.

25. B) Individuals diagnosed with anorexia nervosa tend to be perfectionists and overachievers.

26. D) It is best for the athletic trainer to remain empathetic and calm and help the athlete to see the problem in proportion to the situation so she can deal effectively with the outcome.

27. B) An athlete who threatens suicide must be taken very seriously. It is important to be empathetic and listen to the athlete as he discusses what is troubling him. The team MD should be immediately contacted so that a proper referral to a psychologist or psychiatrist may be made.

Nutrition

1. D) Vitamin A exists in two forms: provitamin A carotenoids (such as dark green and orange vegetables) and preformed vitamin A, which is found in liver, fish oils, fortified milk, and eggs.

2. C) Vitamin C is also known as ascorbic acid. Retinol is vitamin A, and thiamin and niacin are B vitamins.

3. B) Ultraviolet light in sunlight converts a form of cholesterol to vitamin D in the skin.

4. B) During glycolysis, glucose is broken down into pyruvate and ATP. Pyruvate is then broken down into CO_2 and water aerobically or into lactic acid during anaerobic exercise.

5. A) The best time for an athlete to consume carbohydrate-rich food is within 2 hours after training, as glycogen synthesis is the greatest at this time.

6. C) Muscle cells primarily burn fat during low workloads (eg, a brisk walk) because the supply of ATP generated is able to handle that level of work. Intense exercise that may not last more than 30 seconds uses phosphocreatinine and some anaerobic glycolysis to replenish ATP.

7. A) Phosphorus can be found in milk and cheese products, eggs, legumes, nuts, whole grain cereals, meat, fish, and poultry.

8. B) Proteins are long chains of organic compounds called amino acids. There are 22 amino acids, which are used by the body to produce hormones and enzymes. Since the body cannot store excessive protein, some protein is converted into energy or fat.

9. D) Sodium and chloride are electrolytes, which are lost in the greatest amounts while sweating.

10. D) Do not wait for the athlete to complain of being thirsty before supplying fluids. Because the thirst mechanism does not function well when large amounts of fluids are lost by the body during activity, the athlete may need to be reminded to consume fluids frequently.

11. D) The six classes of nutrients include carbohydrates, fats, proteins, water, vitamins, and minerals.

12. C) Water is the most abundant nutrient in the body and must be present in an adequate supply for the body to function normally.

13. C) The new nutrient food label format is known as reference daily intakes (RDI).

14. A) Hydrostatic weighing, electrical impedance, and skin-fold thickness measurements are all means of measuring body composition.

15. B) When more calories are expended than consumed, a negative caloric balance exists and the individual will lose weight.

16. D) Triglyceride, which is a form of fat, is stored in adipose cells and released as the intensity and duration of exercise increases.

17. B) Increasing muscular exercise and dietary intake in appropriate amounts are necessary to increase muscle mass.

18. C) A female athlete who has been diagnosed with a combination of an eating disorder, amenorrhea, and osteoporosis has female triad syndrome.

19. A) Calcium supplements may be necessary to prevent osteoporosis in an athlete who is at high risk for this disease.

20. B) Lactovegetarians eat a diet consisting of plant foods and milk products, but exclude meat products, eggs, and fish. Iron and zinc may be deficient in this diet.

21. A) The body will begin to utilize protein in the event that dietary carbohydrate supply is inadequate.

22. D) Athletes who lack the enzyme lactase have a difficult time digesting dairy products, which causes the development of intestinal gas, diarrhea, and cramping.

23. D) If the body experiences significant electrolyte losses during exercise, the athlete may experience muscular cramping and become susceptible to heat illnesses.

24. A) The kidneys and brain are responsible for regulating water excretion from the body.

25. C) A diet that is significantly lacking in vitamin A will cause poor night vision.

Pharmacology

1. B) Lomotil is an antidiarrheal medication.

2. A) Prozac is a medication used to treat depression, obsessive-compulsive disorder, and bulimia nervosa.

3. D) Pepcid is a medication used to treat heartburn and acid indigestion. It has no stimulant effects.

4. D) Ibuprofen (Advil, Motrin) is available in 200 mg, 400 mg, 600 mg, and 800 mg tablets.

5. B) Diclofenac is known by the brand name Voltaren.

6. A) The recommended dosage for Naprosyn is 250 to 500 mg twice a day.

7. B) An athlete who has overdosed on a stimulant will be agitated and excitable, demonstrate an increase in the respiratory and pulse rates with possible arrhythmias, exhibit tremors, and might become hyperthermic and have convulsions (cocaine affects central thermoregulation) if left untreated.

8. C) Because beta-blockers slow the heart rate, they are potentially performance enhancing during archery.

9. A) Caffeine consumed in moderate amounts will stimulate the cerebral cortex and the medulla, which will increase mental alertness.

10. B) Class I performance-enhancing drugs (which are banned by the IOC) include narcotics, diuretics, and stimulants.

Physics

1. C) The effective radiating area (ERA) is the area of the applicator that emits ultrasound waves to the surface tissue.

2. A) The frequency range of therapeutic ultrasound is between 1.0 to 3.0 MHz.

3. A) The Archimedes principle states that an object immersed in water experiences an upward force that is equal to the weight of the water displaced by the object.

4. B) TENS is a modality for pain relief that is based on the gate control theory.

5. A) A pulsed current during electric stimulation may be monophasic or biphasic.

6. B) The most commonly used frequency used with short-wave diathermy is 27.33 MHz.

7. C) Microwave diathermy produces electromagnetic radiation with a frequency of 2450 megacycles per second and has a wavelength of less than 1 meter.

8. D) There is no "surge" setting on a TENS unit.

9. A) With iontophoresis, ionized medication such as dexamethasone is driven through the skin by a direct electrical current.

10. C) Work equals force times distance.

11. B) Medication delivered by iontophoresis must be ionized.

12. A) According to Joule's law, heat produced by high frequency electrical currents is directly proportional to the square of the current strength, resistance of the conductor, and the time during which the current flows.

13. B) Ohm's law states that the strength of an electric current is equal to the electromotive force divided by the resistance, or $I = V / R$.

14. A) Heat transfers to the skin from a moist heat pack via conduction, which is the transfer of heat by direct contact.

15. C) An alternating current (AC) is an electrical current that reverses direction at a regular interval. A TENS unit utilizes AC current.

16. C) To change a temperature reading from Celsius to Fahrenheit, the following formula must be used: (temperature in Celsius x 9/5) + 32.

17. C) The impedance of a circuit is the resistance that exists within the circuit.

18. C) Moist heat applied during the acute phases of tendinitis will increase pain and enhance the inflammatory process.

19. C) Amperage is the strength of a current flow. It is expressed in amperes.

20. A) According to Poiseille's law, the length and radius of a blood vessel is significant in determining resistance to blood flow.

21. A) Medium-intensity ultrasound is between 0.8 to 1.5 watts per square centimeter.

22. D) The transducer head should be kept between 0.5 to 1 inch from the skin surface during underwater treatment.

23. C) The anode is the positive pole of an electric source.

Administration

1. D) Capital expenses include major costs such as buildings and land. Small supplies such as tape, ultrasound gel, and others used for treatment purposes are direct costs, while office supplies are indirect costs. Staff salaries are not capital costs.

2. D) Changing/locker rooms for the athletes should not be included as a section of the athletic training room.

3. B) An adequately sized training room should be approximately 1000 to 1200 square feet.

4. B) The electrical outlets should be approximately 4 to 5 feet above the floor of the training room with spring-loaded covers to prevent the possibility of electrical shock.

5. A) To maintain confidentiality and security the athletic trainer should utilize a password to prevent unwanted individuals from gaining access to the database.

6. C) The face mask should be located three finger widths from the nose for a correct fit.

7. C) Thermomoldable plastics such as Orthoplast may be used as a hard protective covering for an injured area of the body, such as a dome covering for a quadriceps contusion.

8. C) The NATABOC identified the domains of athletic training as defined by the Role Delineation Study.

9. D) The athletic trainer should keep accurate and up-to-date records in the athletic training room. This information should include items such as injury reports, injury evaluations and progress notes, daily treatment logs, and medical records.

10. C) Line-item budgeting is a method in which the athletic trainer must anticipate the expenditures for specific program functions, such as team physician services, supplies, and equipment repair.

11. B) A certified athletic trainer must acquire 80 CEUs in a 3-year period to maintain certification.

12. D) Licensure is the most restrictive form of regulation for athletic training. Licensure limits the practice of athletic training to those individuals who have successfully met the minimal requirements set by a state licensing board.

13. C) A successful athletic trainer must be an individual who has a love for athletics and competition. He or she must be able to adapt to a variety of environments and deal with diverse personalities of those he or she comes into contact with on a daily basis. The athletic trainer must have a sense of humor and be able to empathize with an athlete who has been injured or is ill. Most importantly, the athletic trainer must be of the highest morals and integrity.

14. D) The school nurse's function in a high school sports medicine program is to act as a liaison between the athletic trainer and the school's health services program.

15. D) The NATA was developed in 1950 to establish practice guidelines and a code of ethics for the athletic training profession.

ANSWER KEY— WRITTEN SIMULATION SAMPLE QUESTIONS

KEY

++ = most appropriate

+ = appropriate, but not first priority

0 = no relevance to the problem

- = not a priority/harmful

-- = detrimental

PROBLEM I

Section A

The current situation: You know that your athlete has been injured as a result of a collision with another soccer player.

Your immediate responsibility: To perform your initial evaluation to determine the type and severity of the injury.

1. +) If the athlete is coherent, it is important for him to identify where there is pain. This gives the athletic trainer an idea of the severity and nature of the injury. (The athlete is awake and complains of neck pain.)

2. --) The athlete should not be moved until a neck or back injury has been ruled out. (The athlete is now a quadriplegic.)

3. ++) This is a quick screen to assess for possible spinal injury. (The athlete can move his fingers and toes.)

4. +) Gathering as much information as possible from those who witnessed the injury is important in understanding how the injury occurred and what the nature of the injury may be. (Another player states he saw the athlete's head "snap" back.)

5. +) As part of a primary survey, it is important to note if there are any bleeding body parts (from a cut or from an orifice). (There is no evidence of bleeding.)

6. 0) Calling an ambulance prior to evaluating this athlete's status would be premature. (The ambulance crew wastes a trip.)

7.   ++) It is necessary to assess the athlete's level of consciousness during the primary survey to determine if there is a life-threatening problem. (The athlete is awake and alert.)

8.   ++) The primary survey is an assessment of any life-threatening problems involving the athlete's airway/breathing, circulation, or severe bleeding. (The athlete's airway is fine, pulse is 80.)

9.   +) If the athlete is conscious and oriented, it is important to have basic knowledge concerning the athlete's prior injuries, especially of the head/neck or back to prevent potential problems even though there may not be any immediate threat to life. (The athlete states he has never had a head injury.)

10. +) The athletic trainer should make a mental note of the athlete's body position in case the athlete must be moved to be treated or transported. (The athlete is lying in supine.)

11. --) Asking the athlete to get up and walk during an initial evaluation is not appropriate until the injury is completely assessed. (The athlete stands and collapses.)

12. +) Checking the pupillary reactions will give the athletic trainer information concerning a possible head injury. (Both pupils react normally.)

13. 0) This action would not be appropriate while performing your initial evaluation on the field. (The athlete wonders why you are placing ice on his shoulder.)

14. --) Unless the athlete is in harm's way while lying on the field, he should not be moved until a complete assessment of his injuries is conducted. (The athlete complains of dizziness and passes out.)

15. +) If the athlete can communicate what occurred, it is important to elicit this information to determine the mechanism and nature of his injury. (The athlete remembers colliding with the other player and felt his head "hit something hard.")

16. +) As part of your primary survey, it is imperative to monitor the athlete's vital signs to detect changes in status. (All vital signs remain stable.)

17. 0) Asking a member of your support team to get a spine board at this time may be a premature action. (The athlete feels okay, is moving, and asks if he is allowed to stand up.)

18. --) The athlete should not be moved until a head, neck, or back injury has been ruled out. (The athlete becomes dizzy.)

Passing mark = 15 questions (correctly answered)

Section B

The current situation: You know that the athlete is conscious and coherent, his vital signs are stable, but he may have sustained a concussion and/or a neck injury.

Your immediate responsibility: Continue with a more indepth evaluation of his neuromuscular function.

19. ++) Once the athlete is on the sidelines, an assessment of his injuries may be conducted in greater detail. (He is able to move his arms but is complaining of left arm "tingling" and a slight headache. There is a small hematoma on his forehead.)

20. ++) It is appropriate to assess the athlete's cognition if there is any evidence of a head injury. (The athlete knows who you are, the date, place, and event.)

21. --) Unless a significant head injury has been completely ruled out, the athlete should be kept awake in order to monitor any changes in level of consciousness. (The athlete becomes lethargic and difficult to arouse.)

22. --) Aspirin has anticoagulant properties; administration of aspirin is contraindicated with a possible head injury. (The athlete has an epidural hematoma and dies.)

23. +) It would be necessary to palpate the cervical area while evaluating the athlete for a possible neck or shoulder injury. (The athlete complains of left upper trapezius soreness.)

24. +) Palpating the trapezius and shoulder girdle musculature may elicit information regarding a musculoskeletal injury to the neck and shoulders. (The athlete is complaining of left-sided neck soreness.)

25. +) This action is a quick screen for the function of C7-T1. (The athlete's left grip strength is weak.)

26. +) The athlete should not return to the game until a secondary survey is complete and the team physician feels confident there are no significant injuries and clears the athlete to play. (A doctor has not examined the athlete yet.)

27. +) Observing the athlete's "body language" will give the athletic trainer an idea of where the injury may be located. (The athlete is holding his left arm.)

28. 0) Assessing the athlete's skin color is not a priority at this time unless the athlete is bleeding severely or the trainer suspects the athlete's circulation may be compromised. (The athlete's skin color is normal.)

29. -) This is not an appropriate action; it does not apply to this situation at this time. (The parents are insulted.)

30. -) The team physician would not need to be notified of the injury at this time unless there was a life-threatening/potentially disabling injury. (The team physician is surprised you do not have the ability to assess the athlete's condition.)

31. -) Calling the athlete's parents would be a premature action. (The parents panic.)

32. 0) This is not an appropriate action; it does not apply to this situation. (The athlete shows no sign of shock.)

33. -) If the athlete can ambulate under his own power without difficulty, he will not need crutches. (There is no evidence of a lower extremity injury.)

Passing mark = 12 questions (correctly answered)

Section C

The current situation: The athlete's vital signs remain stable, and he appears alert and oriented. You suspect the athlete may have sustained a concussion and an upper quarter injury.

Your immediate responsibility: Continue with a detailed examination of the athlete to determine the severity of the injury.

34. 0) Unless there is evidence of a significant problem at this time, monitoring vital signs as frequently as every 10 minutes may or may not be necessary. (The athlete's blood pressure is 120/80, pulse 74 and stable.)

35. +) Manually muscle testing the upper trapezius muscle would be appropriate during your evaluation of this injury. (The athlete can shrug but complains that the left side hurts.)

36. -) An Adson's test is performed when thoracic outlet syndrome is suspected; this athlete has an acute injury. (Review this test and its indications.)

37. +) Manually muscle testing the deltoids would be appropriate during your evaluation of this injury. (The athlete has some difficulty abducting his left arm. Grade = 3/5.)

38. +) Manually muscle testing the rotator cuff musculature would be appropriate during your evaluation of this injury. (The athlete has some difficulty with external rotation of his left arm. Grade = 3+/5.)

39. -) If the athlete has potentially injured his neck or back, this may make the injury worse. If the athlete was feeling lightheaded, it would be better to position him in supine with both legs elevated. (The athlete now has a headache.)

40. -) You have already determined from your sideline evaluation that there is no significant lower extremity injury. A functional movement test is not appropriate at this time. (The athlete is steady while standing and walking.)

41. 0) You have already determined from your sideline evaluation that the athlete is oriented. (The athlete counts backward by increments of seven without difficulty.)

42. +) As part of an upper quarter screen, it may be necessary to check upper extremity deep tendon reflexes. (The left triceps DTR is a little sluggish.)

43. -) The athlete is not in any respiratory distress. (The athlete refuses the mask.)

44. ++) If the physician is available at this time, it would be important for him or her to evaluate the athlete and determine his status for play. (The team physician will arrive in 10 minutes.)

45. --) With a suspected head injury, it would be poor judgment on the athletic trainer's part to allow the athlete to drive. (The athlete gets dizzy and hits a parked car in the parking lot.)

46. +) Checking the sensation of the upper extremities should be included in a detailed evaluation of the athlete in the training room. (There is hypersensitivity in the C7-C8 dermatomes.)

47. +) Checking the range of motion of the athlete's neck should be included in a detailed examination of the athlete. (The athlete has full cervical active range of motion.)

48. -) A positive Tinel's sign is indicative of carpal tunnel syndrome and would be inappropriate, as this was a known traumatic event. (No information is gained from this test.)

49. 0) Palpation of the lateral epicondyle would not provide any helpful information in the evaluation of this athlete. (The athlete states his elbow feels fine.)

50. +) Manually muscle testing the biceps would be appropriate during your evaluation of this injury. (The athlete has some difficulty with resisted elbow flexion. Grade = +3/5.)

51. +) Manually muscle testing the triceps would be appropriate. (The athlete has significant difficulty extending his elbow against resistance. Grade = 3/5.)

Passing mark = 15 questions (correctly answered)

Section D

The current situation: You know that your athlete has sustained a first-degree concussion and a left-sided "burner."

Your immediate responsibility: Monitor the athlete for any changes in his condition and protect the athlete from further harm until he is cleared by the team physician to play.

52. 0) A "burner" is an injury to the nerves of the brachial plexus. An ice pack applied to the upper arm would be ineffective.

53. ++) Persistent sensory changes of the upper extremity would be significant in determining the extent of nerve involvement. (The athlete states his sensation is returning to normal.)

54. -) The athlete has to be cleared by the team doctor in order to return to play. (The athlete returns the next day and is re-injured.)

55. 0) This action would be at the discretion of the physician, not the athletic trainer. (You are reprimanded by your athletic director and team physician.)

56. --) Shoulder strengthening exercises are not indicated with an acute nerve injury. (This action causes further injury to the left upper extremity.)

57. --) This exercise would be contraindicated for an acute upper extremity nerve injury. (The athlete complains of increased pain.)

58. ++) It is prudent to monitor the athlete for a few days after a mild concussion to be sure there is no change in his status. (The athlete's condition returns to normal the next day.)

59. ++) It is imperative that the physician clear the athlete before he returns to full-time activity. (The athlete is cleared to play the second day after the injury.)

60. 0) Giving the athlete a soft neck collar will not cause further injury, but it may not help the athlete either. (The athlete receives a lot of attention by his teammates.)

Passing mark = 7 questions (correctly answered)

PROBLEM II

Section A

The current situation: You know the athlete has sustained a direct blow to the nose causing recurrent nose bleeds.

Your immediate responsibility: Evaluate the athlete for a possible nasal/facial fracture. Stop the bleeding.

1. +) This question is important to ask as part of the history and in understanding the severity of the problem. (The athlete states "he saw stars.")

2. +) Asking whether or not there has been a similar problem in the past is a question that should always be asked when taking a history. (He has had one episode of recurrent nosebleeds 2 years ago from a blow to the nose.)

3. 0) Whether or not the athlete's parents are aware of his nosebleed is irrelevant at this time.

4. 0) Whether or not the athlete has any allergies is insignificant information. (He tells you he is allergic to cats.)

5. -) This action may increase the flow of bleeding. (The bleeding becomes copius.)

6. +) The athlete should be seated in case he becomes faint from the bleeding or pain. (The athlete has no complaints of dizziness.)

7. 0) This action is not necessary in this situation.

8. 0) A noseguard should not be necessary. (This should not be a chronic problem.)

9. --) This action is inappropriate, as heating the area will cause further bleeding. (You have difficulty stopping the bleeding.)

10. 0) It is known from the opening scenario that the origin of this nosebleed was from a blow to the nose, not from chronic high blood pressure.

11. -) Pressure should be applied to the affected nostril, not to the cheek. (This action does nothing to slow the bleeding.)

12. ++) The trainer should palpate the athlete's nose and surrounding areas to be sure no other areas were injured as a result of the earlier trauma (eg, nasal fracture). (The athlete reports tenderness over the bridge of his nose, but there is no crepitus with palpation or deformity.)

13. ++) Swelling with or without deformity may be indicative of a possible nasal fracture. (A small hematoma is noted over the bridge of the nose.)

14. 0) An ice pack placed behind the athlete's neck will be ineffective—it should be placed over the nasal area.

15. --) Under no circumstances should the athlete blow his nose, as this will increase the bleeding. (The bleeding becomes heavy.)

16. ++) Placing a cotton plug under the athlete's top lip will assist in stopping the bleeding. (The bleeding slows down considerably.)

Passing mark = 13 questions (correctly answered)

Section B

The current situation: The athlete has a nosebleed. There is no evidence of a nasal or facial fracture.

Your immediate responsibility: Stop the bleeding.

17. -) This is an unnecessary step at this time. (It is obvious this is not a life-threatening problem.)

18. -) This is an inappropriate step at this time. (The athlete shows no signs of shock.)

19. ++) Having the athlete maintain pressure on the affected nostril will help completely stop the bleeding. (The bleeding stops.)

20. +) It is a prudent step to take, since you will not be following this athlete on a long-term basis. (The coach appreciates your assistance.)

21. -) Most nosebleeds are a minor problem and relatively easy to control. Unless the bleeding cannot be stopped within a 5-minute period, the athlete should be able to return to the competition. (The athlete is furious with you for not allowing him to compete.)

22. 0) This is only necessary if it is determined that this athlete has fractured his nose. (So far there is no indication of a fracture.)

23. -) The athlete should sit upright with his head in a neutral position. (The athlete becomes nauseated from the taste of blood.)

24. -) Calling the visiting team's athletic trainer during your initial treatment is not an appropriate action. (The other athletic trainer wonders why you are calling him during your treatment.)

25. ++) A cotton nose plug soaked with epinephrine hydrochloride will enhance clotting. (The bleeding stops.)

26. --) Aspirin should never be given during active bleeding, as it is an anticoagulant. (The bleeding increases again.)

27. ++) Checking to see that no blood is present on the athlete, his clothing, or the mat and floor are appropriate steps in following universal precautions. (You do a thorough job making sure the blood is cleaned up.)

Passing mark = 9 questions (correctly answered)

Section C

The current situation: The athlete has sustained a nosebleed secondary to a traumatic blow to the nose, which is beginning to resolve.

Your immediate responsibility: Stop the bleeding and return the athlete to competition.

28. -) As long as the nosebleed has been brought under control, it is not necessary to call your team doctor. (The doctor is upset you wasted time calling him.)

29. --) It is not your place to call the visiting team's doctor regarding a minor nosebleed. (This physician thinks you are incompetent.)

30. 0) This action may only serve to unnecessarily alarm the athlete and his parents and should only be initiated if the nose needs to be cauterized by a doctor. (You panic the parents.)

31. -) There is no reason to restrict this athlete's fluid intake. (The athlete becomes dehydrated.)

32. ++) As long as the bleeding has completely stopped, the athlete can return to competition. (He wins his match.)

33. -) This is an unnecessary action if no swelling or deformity of the nose is evident, as the bleeding has stopped. (The team physician is upset that you suggested this.)

34. ++) It would be a responsible step to contact the athlete's home athletic trainer to report the incident and what treatment was administered. (The athletic trainer appreciates your information.)

35. --) Sit-ups temporarily increase blood pressure and capillary pressure, which may produce another spontaneous nosebleed. (The athlete's nose begins bleeding again.)

36. ++) Biohazard bags should be used as a universal precaution. (The athletic director appreciates you following protocol.)

37. +) The athlete should be monitored during the competition for any further problems. (The athlete has no further episodes of bleeding.)

38. +) The athlete should keep an ice pack on his nose while he is not competing to minimize pain and encourage clotting. (He reports the pain and swelling have decreased.)

Passing mark = 9 questions (correctly answered)

PROBLEM III

Section A

The current situation: You know your athlete has injured his right lower leg during a dismount off the rings.

Your immediate responsibility: To perform your initial evaluation to determine the type and severity of the injury.

1. ++) Since this injury was not witnessed, information should be obtained from the athlete about what occurred as part of the "history" portion of the initial evaluation. (The athlete tells you he was not balanced and landed on his right side.)

2. ++) Because the opening scene has implied there is a significant lower extremity injury, the athletic trainer should ask the athlete if he heard/felt a "snap" or "pop," which may indicate a ligament injury or fracture. (The athlete definitely felt a "snap.")

3. ++) This will give the athletic trainer an idea of the athlete's willingness to move his leg. (The athlete won't move his leg because of pain.)

4. +) Observing for areas of swelling and/or bleeding is part of a secondary survey. (The distal lower extremity is swollen with deformity.)

5. +) Palpation of the injured area is part of the secondary survey. (The athlete has significant pain with palpation of the lower leg.)

6. ++) Because this appears to be a significant injury, it would be prudent for the athletic trainer to monitor the athlete's vital signs. (Blood pressure is 128/88 and pulse of 88.)

7. ++) The pulses of the lower leg should be assessed to make sure there is adequate circulation to the affected limb. (The right popliteal pulse is palpable and strong.)

8. --) Heating the affected area is contraindicated during the acute phase of the injury. (The effusion becomes enormous.)

9. -) The injured leg should not be moved until your initial evaluation is complete. (The athlete screams in pain.)

10. +) It has been determined this injury is serious enough to warrant calling for an ambulance.

11. -) It has been determined that there is a significant injury to the right lower extremity. It is not necessary to spend a lot of time examining the athlete's entire body for injuries. (A lot of time has been wasted.)

12. +) If the area that is injured is not immediately accessible, it may be necessary to cut away the athlete's uniform. (You can clearly see where the injury is located.)

13. 0) Until the severity of the injury is established, immobilization of the limb may be a premature action.

Passing mark = 10 questions (correctly answered)

Section B

The current situation: The athlete is complaining of severe right lower leg pain; the lower leg is swollen and obviously deformed. The athlete's vital signs are stable.

Your immediate responsibility: Continue your evaluation, then stabilize the leg and make the athlete comfortable.

14. --) If a fracture is suspected, the athletic trainer should never manipulate the injured area, as this will cause further injury. (The deformity is worsened.)

15. -) The athlete should not be moved until the immobilizer or splint is in place and secured on the affected limb. (The athlete screams in pain.)

16. 0) This action would only be necessary if a crowd is gathering and/or there is equipment that is in the way.

17. +) This action is appropriate to decrease pain and minimize effusion. (The athlete feels better with ice on his leg.)

18. ++) It is critical to check the pulses of the ankle and foot to determine if there is adequate circulation to the injured limb. (The right dorsalis pedis pulse is palpable, but weak.)

19. ++) If the leg appears hard and swollen, it may indicate the beginning of a Volkmann's contracture, which is a paralytic contracture that results from ischemia of muscles and nerves in an extremity. (The lower leg appears tight and swollen.)

20. 0) The competition should be stopped if the athlete is in harm's way or an entrance/exit to the gym area is blocked because of crowding.

21. --) Moving the athlete may cause further injury; initial immobilization should take place with the athlete in sidelying position. (The deformity is made worse by moving the leg.)

22. -) It has been determined by this time that the athlete has a significant lower leg injury. Evaluating the hip at this time is both unnecessary and inappropriate. (You wasted valuable time.)

23. +) Assuming the leg is immobilized at this point, short-term elevation may help retard swelling.

24. -) Checking for crepitus at this time is inappropriate. (The athlete screams in pain.)

25. ++) If a fracture is suspected of the lower extremity, immobilization is a priority in preventing further injury. (The leg is immobilized while the athlete is in sidelying.)

26. --) Massaging the area of injury is inappropriate and will cause increased pain and swelling. (The athlete screams in pain.)

Passing mark = 10 questions (correctly answered)

Section C

The current situation: You have determined the athlete has sustained a lower leg fracture. The athlete's leg is immobilized.

Your immediate responsibility: Prepare to transport the athlete to the hospital and monitor the athlete until the rescue squad arrives. Document the event and your actions.

27. +) This is an appropriate action to assess circulation and neurological function. (The athlete complains his foot feels numb.)

28. --) This action would be inappropriate. The athlete should be transported by a gurney to minimize movement of the lower body. (The athlete trips with the crutches.)

29. --) Issuing any medications to this athlete would not be appropriate action at this point in time because it is unknown what other medications he will be given at the hospital. (The team physician finds out and is furious.)

30. -) It is not necessary for the coach to accompany this athlete to the hospital. It is the duty of the athletic trainer to follow up with this athlete after the meet is finished. (A parent substitutes for the coach and the team loses.)

31. --) It is unknown what the athlete will be given at the hospital (medications, etc) or if he may need anesthesia. It is dangerous to allow the athlete to eat or drink as he wants until he is told it is okay by the medical staff at the hospital. (The athlete aspirates in the operating room and dies.)

32. -) It is unknown what this athlete's status is at this time and the decision to return to play will be up to the team physician. (The coach wants to know if you spoke with the team physician.)

33. 0) If the trainer has a personal rapport with the emergency room staff, this is a nice touch, but not necessary. The rescue squad will alert the hospital of their arrival. (The emergency room nurse politely thanks you for your call.)

34. ++) Monitoring the athlete for symptoms of shock is always appropriate with a traumatic injury and your findings should be passed along to the EMS team. (The athlete appears pale and his blood pressure has dropped to 90/60 with a pulse rate of 90.)

35. ++) It is important that the athletic trainer emotionally support the athlete. Realize he is in pain and scared and will need reassurance that he is in good hands. (The athlete is calm with your presence.)

36. 0) Fitting the athlete for a pair of crutches is unnecessary. (The hospital will handle it.)

37. +) If this athlete is a minor, his parents should be contacted and given information on what occurred, what actions were taken to care for the athlete, and to which hospital he was sent. (The parents leave for the hospital and are grateful you called.)

38. +) An injury report should be filled out to ensure the circumstances surrounding the injury and what steps were taken during his care are documented. (You avoid a potential malpractice lawsuit.)

Passing mark = 10 questions (correctly answered)

PROBLEM IV

Section A

The current situation: You know your athlete has injured his left ankle.

Your immediate responsibility: To perform your initial evaluation to determine the nature and severity of the injury.

1. -) You witnessed the injury. It is obvious that his left ankle is involved, not his back. Evaluating this athlete's low back is unnecessary. (The athlete thinks you are incompetent.)

2. -) It is obvious from the information given in the opening scenario that the athlete is able to bear weight on the ankle without assistance. Getting a wheelchair is inappropriate. (The athlete wonders for whom you are getting a wheelchair.)

3. 0) This is an unnecessary action. It has been determined that the athlete has injured his left ankle. (Now the athlete definitely does not trust you.)

4. +) It is important to make a bilateral comparison of both ankles when observing for swelling, ecchymosis, or deformity during the initial evaluation. (The left ankle is swollen on the lateral side.)

5. --) This is an inappropriate action and may cause further injury. (The athlete re-injures his ankle.)

6. --) This is an unnecessary and inappropriate action and may cause further injury. (The pain and swelling increase.)

7. -) A Lachman's test is not a special test for the ankle. (The athlete's knees are fine.)

8. +) An anterior drawer test should be performed bilaterally to determine if there is any ankle joint instability. (There is a positive result on the left ankle.)

9. ++) Palpation is an integral portion of the initial evaluation. (There is tenderness over the ATF and CF ligaments.)

10. ++) Checking the athlete's willingness to move is an integral segment of the initial evaluation. Comparing the active range of motion of the involved joint to the uninvolved side is a necessary step in an orthopedic assessment. (The athlete complains of pain with active movement into dorsiflexion and eversion.)

Passing mark = 8 questions (correctly answered)

Section B

The current situation: The athlete has a grade II inversion sprain of the left ankle with injury to the anterior talofibular and calcaneofibular ligament.

Your immediate responsibility: To begin treating the injury to reduce the pain and swelling.

11. ++) During the acute stages of treatment, the athlete should be kept in nonweight-bearing or partial weight-bearing to minimize pain and swelling. (There is less pain in nonweight-bearing.)

12. -) Although aspirin is an anti-inflammatory with analgesic properties, it would be contraindicated at this time because it may cause further bleeding into the joint. (The swelling increases.)

13. ++) Rest, ice, compression, and elevation are primary components of the initial treatment of an acute musculoskeletal injury. (The pain and swelling decrease.)

14. 0) Calling the team doctor at this time is unnecessary and inappropriate. (The doctor wonders why you don't know how to treat an acute ankle sprain.)

15. --) Ultrasound is a deep-heating modality. This is a definite "no-no" during the acute stage of treatment. (The pain and swelling increase significantly.)

16. --) As with ultrasound, a warm or hot whirlpool will only make the pain and swelling worse. (The ankle is very swollen.)

17. +) Keeping the athlete in nonweight-bearing at this time is proper protocol in the immediate care of an acute injury. (The athlete is able to ambulate comfortably with crutches.)

18. 0) Unless you suspect a more significant injury at this point, this action is inappropriate. (The athlete has not seen a doctor.)

19. 0) The immediate care of an acute ankle sprain does not include upper body reconditioning.

20. +) It is the athletic trainer's duty to keep the athlete's coach well-informed about the athlete's injury and treatment. (He appreciates your report.)

21. -) Resistive ankle strengthening exercises would be inappropriate at this time. (The ankle is too weak and the pain is increased with resistance.)

Passing mark = 9 questions (correctly answered)

Section C

The current situation: You have determined the athlete has sustained a grade II inversion sprain with injury to the anterior talofibular ligament and calcaneofibular ligament. Treatment has been initiated to reduce the pain and swelling.

Your immediate responsibility: To ensure the athlete knows how to care for his injury at home.

22. -) Although going to the emergency room would not hurt the athlete, it may not be necessary either. (The athlete spends 3 hours in the emergency room to be diagnosed with a sprain.)

23. 0) It is courteous to contact the parents if the athlete is a minor, but this may be an unnecessary step. (The athlete is able to follow your instructions overnight.)

24. --) Closed-chain exercises would be contraindicated with such an acute ankle injury. (The ankle pain increases.)

25. ++) This is a fundamental component of treatment of an acute musculoskeletal injury. (The pain and swelling are controlled.)

26. +) This is a fundamental component of treatment of an acute musculoskeletal injury. (The swelling is controlled.)

27. 0) Wearing high-top sneakers will not change the athlete's condition. (Although they look "cool.")

28. --) Attempting to hop on an acutely injured ankle is inappropriate and will cause further injury to an already traumatized joint. (The athlete falls and sprains his ankle again.)

Passing mark = 6 questions (correctly answered)

PROBLEM V

Section A

The current situation: You know your athlete has sustained a traumatic injury to her eyes and/or face as a result of a blow by a hockey ball.

Your immediate responsibility: To perform your initial evaluation to determine the nature and severity of the injury.

1. 0) With the exception of the goalie, there is no head/face protective equipment in field hockey.

2. -) From the information provided by the opening scenario, you know the athlete has an eye and/or facial injury. Testing the athlete's fine motor skills is inappropriate. (There is no problem with the athlete's fine motor skills.)

3. -) It has been determined that this is an injury to the eye and/or face. Attempting to test this athlete's balance is inappropriate. (The athlete wonders why you want her to balance on one leg.)

4. --) The use of an ammonia capsule would be unnecessary and inappropriate. The athlete may jerk her head, possibly causing further injury. (The athlete sustains a retinal detachment.)

5. --) This athlete may have a potentially serious eye injury. The athlete should remain in a recumbent position until the initial injury assessment is complete. (The athlete complains of "throbbing" pain.)

6. +) This is an appropriate action but does not directly relate to your evaluation. (The athlete is more comfortable.)

7. 0) Asking the athlete who made the shot is an inappropriate question. (Who cares?)

8. +) This is an appropriate question during an injury assessment as part of the "subjective" information portion of the evaluation. (The athlete complains of pain above the right eye.)

9. 0) Although examining the shoulders will not harm the athlete, it has been determined the injury is to the eye. (The athlete has no shoulder pain.)

10. ++) It is important the athletic trainer perform a primary survey and thoroughly examine the head, face, or neck as indicated once the mechanism of injury has been determined. (It is determined this is not a life-threatening situation.)

11. ++) Gently palpating the orbital rim and nose for point tenderness, crepitus, or deformity is part of the initial assessment of an eye injury. (There is tenderness over the left eyebrow with a large hematoma. No crepitus is noted.)

12. ++) Because this was a traumatic injury involving a small high-velocity projectile, it is highly likely blood will be present. (Donning gloves is part of universal precautions.)

13. -) A "battle sign" is present when there is a basilar skull fracture. It is known from the opening scene that the athlete has suffered an eye injury.

14. 0) Asking the athlete if she is a scholarship athlete is unnecessary and inappropriate. (The athlete asks why that matters.)

15. ++) Checking the area for bleeding is a fundamental component of your initial examination of this athlete. (There is a profuse amount of blood present.)

16. +) This is an appropriate question when assessing the severity of injury to the eye itself. (The athlete's vision is blurred.)

Passing mark = 13 questions (correctly answered)

Section B

The current situation: You know the athlete has a deep laceration above the left eyebrow. It does not appear that the athlete has sustained any facial fractures.

Your immediate responsibility: To clean and dress the wound and treat the athlete for pain and swelling.

17. ++) It is important to check pupillary response for possible cerebral injury. (The pupillary response is normal.)

18. --) This would be contradicted in an acute injury to the eye. (The bleeding and swelling increase dramatically.)

19. +) Rinsing the wound with saline solution will help to remove any dirt or debris that may cause an infection.

20. 0) Because this is a deep laceration, the athlete will have to be referred to a physician for treatment. Application of an antiseptic or antibiotic to the area after a thorough cleansing will be done by the physician.

21. +) Both eyes should be covered during the athlete's transport to the hospital to minimize eye movement. (The athlete feels better with her eyes closed.)

22. 0) The mechanism of injury was determined by the opening scenario. (This is obvious.)

23. +) Because there is no apparent injury to the eye itself, an ice pack applied lightly to the surrounding area of the eye will help minimize swelling. (The pain and swelling are controlled.)

24. +) The application of Steri-strips will help to minimize bleeding and approximate the wound until the physician sutures it. (You are able to close the wound.)

25. -) It is inappropriate to ignore the athlete. It is the job of the athletic trainer to answer her questions honestly and be reassuring to minimize her anxieties. (The athlete appears fearful.)

26. --) Only a physician can suture a wound; an athletic trainer is not qualified or licensed to do so. (You are sued for malpractice.)

27. +) If there is a suspected serious eye injury, the athlete should be transported to a hospital while lying in a recumbent position. (You act cautiously.)

28. --) The athlete should be kept calm and comfortable while waiting for the ambulance and should not be left alone. (The athlete passes out in the parking lot.)

29. -) In case of a serious eye injury, no direct pressure should be applied to the eye. (You find out later you might have made the injury worse.)

30. ++) A secondary evaluation is a detailed assessment that focuses on the nature and extent of the injury. (You know the athlete has a bad laceration and suspect a potentially serious eye injury.)

Passing mark = 11 questions (correctly answered)

Section C

The current situation: The athlete has sustained a deep laceration over the left eyebrow with a potential eye injury.

Your immediate responsibility: Keep the athlete calm while waiting for the rescue squad and document the course of events.

31. +) The athletic trainer should be a source of reassurance. This is an appropriate action. (The athlete is grateful you are staying with her.)

32. -) The athlete's condition and playing status have not been determined. Announcing the athlete's condition is inappropriate. (You anger the coach and parents with this announcement.)

33. -) The student's insurance coverage should not be a deterrent for an emergency room visit. (You delay treatment.)

34. -) It is not the duty of the school nurse to accompany the athlete to the emergency room. (She reminds you that this is part of your job.)

35. --) Once the initial dressing is applied and the bleeding is controlled, it is inappropriate to change the bandage multiple times. (The Steri-strips come off and the cut bleeds again.)

36. +) The athlete may need reassurance from her coach that her position is not in jeopardy. (The coach tells the athlete there is no need to worry.)

37. -) Speaking with the press about the athlete's condition is not appropriate. (You are reprimanded by your athletic director.)

38. ++) Washing your hands thoroughly after handling a "blood-spill" is a fundamental universal precaution.

39. ++) Documenting the incident and treatment given is appropriate.

40. 0) Dispensing vitamins to the athlete is unnecessary and inappropriate.

41. +) Once the athlete is stable and not in any immediate danger, it is wise to inform the athlete's coach on the nature and severity of the injury and what is being done for her. (The coach thanks you for doing a thorough job.)

Passing mark = 9 questions (correctly answered)

Problem VI

Section A

The current situation: You have been made aware of an athlete who may have a serious eating disorder.

Your immediate responsibility: Educate and advise the coach not to encourage her current behavior, but to emphasize the importance of proper nutritional habits and to keep the athletic training staff informed of her behavior.

1. --) Because anorexia nervosa is an eating disorder that is characterized by a distorted body image and is caused by a deep-seated and complex interaction of psychological and sociocultural factors, the athlete must be gently confronted and not attacked. Unless the athlete is in immediate danger, threatening the athlete is inappropriate. (The athlete is so upset, she quits the team.)

2. +) Continual fixation on the athlete's weight changes in relation to her athletic performance may encourage destructive behavior.

3. 0) Keeping a diary of the time or place the athlete eats is unnecessary. Treatment should be implemented by those qualified to do so, such as a psychologist or physician. (The coach wastes a lot of paper.)

4. +) Emphasizing the importance of good nutritional habits in optimizing athletic performance is an appropriate action. (The athlete seems to respond in a positive manner and begins eating a small, but regular breakfast.)

5. ++) Any behavior(s) associated with eating disorders that become prominent must be relayed to the athletic training staff so the athlete can be immediately referred for professional help. (You are able to provide the team physician with valuable information.)

Passing mark = 4 questions (correctly answered)

Section B

The current situation: You have identified an athlete who has an eating disorder and you have advised the coach how to properly handle the situation.

Your immediate responsibility: Continue to monitor the athlete's behavior and educate and support the athlete.

6. +) Providing constructive advice is an appropriate action. (The athlete agrees to try to reach the set goals.)

7. -) Using an approach that threatens the athlete in any fashion is not appropriate. (The athlete feels challenged and continues to abuse laxatives anyway.)

8. +) Encouraging the athlete to express her feelings is an important and necessary step in her recovery. (She states she feels her parents won't love her if she is not the best gymnast on the team.)

9. 0) Addressing the issue with the athletic director is not necessary. (He tells you to discuss the matter with your team doctor.)

10. -) To make the assumption that the athlete will be removed from the team is premature and is ultimately a decision that will be made by the coach. (The athlete panics.)

11. --) It is not wise to make promises that you may not be able to keep. If this athlete is seriously ill, the coach may cut her from the team. (The coach is debating what to do.)

12. -) This athlete will need the support of the coaching and athletic training staff to actively seek professional counseling. (The athlete does not have the self-esteem to initiate counseling on her own.)

13. ++) The athlete needs to be gently confronted with specific behaviors that the coach and athletic trainer have observed to move the athlete toward recovery. (The athlete admits she has a problem.)

Passing mark = 6 questions (correctly answered)

Section C

The current situation: You have identified an athlete with a significant eating disorder. The athlete acknowledges she has a problem.

Your immediate responsibility: Make sure the athlete is referred to a psychologist for treatment.

14. ++) The team physician needs to be aware of the problem to arrange for psychological or psychiatric treatment. (The team doctor tells you he will make a referral to a psychiatrist.)

15. 0) This is an appropriate action but should occur in conjunction with the team physician.

16. -) Anorexia nervosa and bulimia are primarily psychological disorders. Placing the athlete on a diet intended to encourage weight gain will not be enough to solve this problem. (She follows the diet for 2 days.)

17. 0) Weighing the athlete will not have an impact on changing her behavior at this time.

18. --) The athletic trainer is not qualified to arrange for this type of intervention. (The team doctor is very upset with your actions.)

19. -) This would be an inappropriate referral for this athlete. (The sports nutritionist reminds you she does not have a degree in psychology.)

20. 0) Although having the athlete eat these foods would not hurt her, she is likely not to comply. She needs professional psychological treatment, so this action would not be appropriate. (This athlete is a vegetarian and hates bananas.)

Passing mark = 6 questions (correctly answered)

PROBLEM VII

Section A

The current situation: You know your athlete has been injured after incorrectly landing on a crash mat. He is not moving.

Your immediate responsibility: To evaluate the injury to determine the type and nature of the injury.

1. -) This would be a premature action as you have not completed your initial evaluation of the injury.

2. +) This question should be asked as part of the "history" portion of the initial assessment. (The athlete complains of dull neck pain.)

3. ++) A primary survey is necessary to determine if there is a life-threatening injury. (The athlete is conscious and is breathing without difficulty. Blood pressure is 130/90 and pulse is 82.)

4. +) Noting the position of the athlete is important when deciding how the athlete is to be treated and transported. (The athlete is lying on his right side with his knees flexed.)

5. -) The athlete should not be moved unless the airway is blocked and there is additional help available. (The athlete is breathing without difficulty.)

6. +) This is a quick screen to assess motor function of the upper and lower extremities. (The athlete states he cannot move his fingers or toes.)

7. +) If the athlete is conscious and can answer questions, it is appropriate to ask this as part of the history portion of the evaluation. It helps in determining the mechanism of injury. (He reports he did not tuck his chin in and landed on his head, snapping his head forward.)

8. 0) Applying an ice pack to the athlete's neck is unnecessary and inappropriate.

9. 0) It is known from the opening scenario that the area of injury is not the lower extremity.

10. +) It is an appropriate action as part of the primary survey to assess the athlete for areas of significant bleeding. (The athlete's face in uninjured.)

11. 0) Until the initial evaluation of the injury is completed, this would be a premature and inappropriate action. (You waste valuable time.)

12. ++) Checking the athlete's level of consciousness is a necessary step during the primary survey. (The athlete is coherent and responds appropriately to questions.)

Passing mark = 10 questions (correctly answered)

Section B

The current situation: The athlete is conscious and coherent and is breathing without difficulty. His vital signs are stable, but he is unable to move his extremities.

Your immediate responsibility: To continue your evaluation to determine the athlete's neuromuscular function, protect the athlete from further injury and prepare him for transport to the hospital.

13. --) Moving the athlete at this time without securing him to a spine board may cause further injury. (The athlete sustains a complete spinal cord injury and is quadriplegic.)

14. --) Having the athlete move his head may be a potentially fatal or debilitating action. (The athlete sustained a vertebral fracture/dislocation and dies.)

15. ++) Determining sensation to the extremities is important in assessing the severity of the injury. (The athlete complains he cannot feel anything from his armpits down to his feet.)

16. ++) This is a fundamental action in preventing further injury to the athlete.

17. 0) This is an unnecessary action, as you have ruled out a head injury. (The athlete is conscious and alert.)

18. -) The findings of the primary survey do not indicate there is a head injury. (You waste time.)

19. ++) Log-rolling the athlete with assistance onto his back is necessary for stabilization and transport of the athlete. (You successfully position the athlete into supine.)

20. 0) Unless the athlete is in an area where he may be subjected to further injury, it is not necessary to stop the meet at this time. (You keep the area clear of spectators.)

21. ++) Securing the athlete to a spine board is an appropriate action. (You successfully secure the athlete onto a spine board with help.)

22. ++) While you stay with the athlete, an ambulance should be summoned to the field. (The ambulance is close by and arrives in 5 minutes.)

23. +) This is an appropriate action with a suspected neck injury. (You successfully apply a cervical collar.)

24. +) Monitoring the athlete's vital signs is a fundamental aspect of your care. (The athlete's vital signs remain stable.)

Passing mark = 10 questions (correctly answered)

Section C

The current situation: You have evaluated the injury and suspect the athlete has sustained a serious cervical spinal injury. The athlete is transported to the hospital via ambulance.

Your immediate responsibility: To contact the team physician, parents, and other appropriate individuals with information regarding the accident. Document what occurred and who was involved.

25. +) Communicating with the team physician would be appropriate at this time. (Your student trainer contacts the team doctor's office.)

26. +) It is important to document the incident. (You protect yourself against a malpractice lawsuit.)

27. 0) If another certified athletic trainer is available to cover the rest of the meet, it would be appropriate to go to the hospital. Otherwise, you should follow up with the athlete at the hospital after the meet.

28. 0) The athlete is coherent and able to provide this information to the EMS and hospital personnel.

29. 0) Whether or not the athlete is on a scholarship is not pertinent to the treatment of this athlete.

30. +) Contacting the parents of the injured athlete would be an appropriate step. (The parents go directly to the hospital.)

31. -) Leaving a student athletic trainer in charge of covering a state track meet without direct supervision of a certified athletic trainer is inappropriate. (You are reprimanded by your athletic director and are lucky no one else is hurt while you are gone.)

32. -) This is an inappropriate comment. (The athletic director suggests that you stick to your duties as an athletic trainer.)

Passing mark = 6 questions (correctly answered)

Problem VIII

Section A

The current situation: An athlete comes to your office complaining of chronic left anterior knee pain. No specific mechanism of injury has been identified.

Your immediate responsibility: To perform your initial evaluation to determine the nature and severity of the condition.

1. 0) Applying an ice pack will not cause further injury, but may not help the athlete either, because the problem has not been thoroughly evaluated at this time.

2. +) A postural assessment is part of the evaluation of anterior knee pain. (Both knees are in genu valgum.)

3. +) Palpation of the knee joint is a basic element of a knee evaluation. (The athlete complains of patellar tendon and medial knee pain.)

4. +) With subjective complaints of anterior knee pain, it is highly likely the athlete's iliotibial band will be tight. Both sides must be tested for comparison. (Ober test is positive on the left lower extremity.)

5. +) This question should be asked while taking the athlete's history, as a "popping" sensation is often associated with patellofemoral pain syndrome. (The athlete reports it "pops" intermittently while running.)

6. -) It is known from the athlete's subjective complaints that this is a knee injury. (The athlete tells you her feet are fine.)

7. 0) A Patrick's test is a special test of the hip which, when positive, is indicative of degenerative joint disease.

8. +) This is an appropriate question to ask when gathering information regarding the mechanism of injury. (The athlete has pain going down stairs and running downhill.)

9. ++) Because activity appears to increase the pain, it would be wise to advise the athlete to stop running when it hurts. (The athlete feels much better when she is not landing on it.)

10. -) Temporary orthotics may not be necessary or appropriate; the initial evaluation is not complete. (You waste time making them and the athlete reports no change in her pain.)

11. +) Observing the knee for swelling or deformity is a fundamental component of the initial evaluation. (No swelling is noted.)

12. +) Palpating the knee joint and surrounding soft tissue structures is a fundamental component of the initial evaluation. (The athlete complains of pain with palpation of the medial facet.)

13. -) A KT-1000 arthrometer is used to test for anterior cruciate laxity and would not be appropriate in this situation. (It is known from the opening scenario that this is not an acute injury and injury to the anterior cruciate ligament is unlikely.)

Passing mark = 10 questions (correctly answered)

Section B

The current situation: The athlete has pain running downhill, especially over the patellar tendon and medial aspect of the knee. She has pain over the same areas with palpation, although there is no swelling present. She also experiences a "popping" sensation with running. She stands in genu valgum and presents a tight iliotibial band on the left leg.

Your immediate responsibility: Make recommendations to the athlete to decrease her pain with activities and teach the athlete lower limb stretching and strengthening exercises to realign the patella.

14. +) A soft knee brace designed to help stabilize the patella may help decrease the athlete's pain during activity. (The athlete reports a decrease in pain and feeling of "popping" while wearing the knee sleeve.)

15. 0) Strengthening the hamstrings does not have a direct effect in stabilizing the patella.

16. +) Strengthening the vastus medialis obliquis will help to improve the tracking of the patella in the femoral groove. (The athlete has fewer episodes of "popping.")

17. --) Repetitive deep squatting exercises cause high compressive loading on the patellofemoral joint and will aggravate the athlete's knee. (The athlete complains of significant anterior knee pain.)

18. +) Patella taping is a useful tool in evaluating and treating patellar misalignment problems. (There is reduction of pain with taping.)

19. ++) A tight iliotibial band will cause mistracking of the patella. (There are fewer episodes of popping.)

20. ++) Tight hamstrings may cause mistracking of the patella in the femoral groove. (The athlete has bilateral hamstring tightness.)

21. -) Recommending an oral NSAID might be appropriate, but a certified athletic trainer is not qualified or licensed to dispense a prescription drug such as Voltaren. (The athlete has an adverse reaction to the medication and you are sued for malpractice.)

22. -) The athlete should avoid hard or hilly surfaces. (The athlete continues to complain of "popping" and knee pain with running.)

Passing mark = 7 questions (correctly answered)

Section C

The current situation: You have determined from your evaluation that this athlete has a subluxing patella secondary to weak anteromedial thigh musculature and a tight iliotibial band and hamstrings.

Your immediate responsibility: Continue to work with the athlete to develop a structured rehabilitation program to encourage proper alignment of the patella, which will in turn eliminate the pain.

23. 0) A TENS unit is a modality that can be used temporarily for pain. A TENS unit will not contribute directly to the elimination of the origin of the problem. (The athlete has no pain when she is not running.)

24. -) The patella subluxes as a result of weak anterior and medial thigh musculature; PNF exercises that emphasize motions which encourage hip abduction with internal rotation facilitate strengthening of the lateral thigh musculature. (The athlete experiences an increase in episodes of patella subluxation.)

25. 0) Ultrasound treatments will not have a direct impact on the cause of the problem.

26. --) Because plyometric exercises employ ballistic movements, which generate high forces, the initiation of this type of exercise would not be appropriate. (The athlete now complains of anterior knee pain at rest.)

27. ++) Strengthening the quadriceps musculature in both open- and closed-chain positions is appropriate as long as the exercise is pain-free.

28. +) It may be beneficial to evaluate the athlete's running gait to assess what is occurring at the knee. (The athlete's feet severely pronate during midstance.)

29. ++) Strengthening the hip adductors will augment the strength of the vastus medialis oblique muscle.

30. +) The continual application of ice to the knee will help minimize any pain or inflammation from exercises. (The athlete is able to control post-activity soreness.)

Passing mark = 6 questions (correctly answered)

PROBLEM IX

Section A

The current situation: Your athlete presents to you with abdominal cramping and diarrhea of unknown origin, which has lasted 2 days.

Your immediate responsibility: To try to identify the etiology of the problem and perform an initial evaluation to determine the extent of the problem.

1. ++) It is important to evaluate what types of food and drink the athlete has consumed because certain foods (such as spicy foods) may lead to dyspepsia or diarrhea. (The athlete states he has not eaten any spicy foods.)

2. +) Anxiety can contribute to gastrointestinal upset. This is an appropriate question to ask the athlete during the history portion of your initial assessment. (The athlete admits he is nervous.)

3. ++) This is an appropriate question to ask during the history portion of the initial evaluation because it will help to identify if the athlete has an underlying gastrointestinal problem. (The athlete states this frequently happens at the beginning of the season.)

4. 0) This action would be appropriate if you suspect the athlete is dehydrated. (The athlete complains his lips feel dry, but he is not excessively thirsty. Blood pressure 115/70.)

5. +) This is an appropriate action because the athlete might have a fever secondary to an infection. (The athlete's oral temperature is within normal limits.)

6. 0) This is an inappropriate action. It does not directly relate to the athlete's condition.

7. 0) This is an unnecessary and inappropriate action. (The athlete complains of "gas pain" with palpation of his abdomen.)

8. --) Running or increased activity will only contribute to gastrointestinal upset and is an inappropriate action at this point. It will not provide any information regarding the cause of the problem (The athlete has a severe episode of diarrhea after running).

Passing mark = 6 questions (correctly answered)

Section B

The current situation: You have determined that the athlete has developed gastrointestinal upset because of precompetition anxiety.

Your immediate responsibility: Treat for abdominal cramping, diarrhea, and prevent dehydration.

9. +) If the athlete is very uncomfortable and is feeling "weak," this would be an appropriate action to take. (The athlete feels better at rest.)

10. ++) This would be an appropriate action to monitor the athlete for degree of dehydration. (The athlete loses 3 pounds after a strenuous workout.)

11. ++) An over-the-counter antimotility medication such as Imodium or Peptobismol may reduce the cramping and diarrhea. (The athlete responds well to this and the diarrhea stops.)

12. -) Certain vegetables may cause intestinal gas formation and would be inappropriate to add to the athlete's diet at this time.

13. --) It would be best to give the athlete clear fluids. Milk may cause nausea and increased flatulence; soda and tea contain caffeine, which has a diuretic effect. (The athlete becomes significantly dehydrated.)

14. 0) This would be an inappropriate action. Only one of your athletes is complaining of gastrointestinal distress. (The hotel management finds out what you are doing and is outraged.)

15. 0) Although this is not necessary, drinking bottled water will not be harmful to the athlete.

Passing mark = 6 questions (correctly answered)

PROBLEM X

Section A

The current situation: You know your athlete has injured his right knee while playing soccer and he is only able to partially bear weight on the involved limb.

Your immediate responsibility: To perform your initial evaluation to determine the type and severity of the injury.

1. +) Palpating the joint and the surrounding soft tissue structures is an appropriate action during the initial evaluation of the injury. (The athlete is significantly tender over the anteriomedial joint line and the medial retinaculum.)

2. --) Performing a functional movement such as a deep squat is inappropriate during the initial assessment. (The athlete refuses to do this.)

3. ++) Since you were not present during the actual injury, you must rely on the athlete's account of what occurred to determine the mechanism of injury. (The athlete reports feeling a "pop" and sharp knee pain after planting his right leg to kick the ball with his left leg.)

4. +) It is an appropriate action to check the circulation of the injured limb distal to the injury site. (The circulation is fine.)

5. +) This is an appropriate question to ask during the history portion of the evaluation. (The athlete has told you he felt a "pop.")

6. -) This is an inappropriate test for a knee injury. A Speed's test is used to assess for the presence of bicipital tendinitis.

7. ++) Based on information given in the opening scenario and the mechanism of injury, this would be an appropriate special test to perform. (The Lachman's test is positive on the right knee.)

8. 0) Although this was a traumatic incident, there was no direct insult. Crepitus would be present with a possible fracture or a chronic problem such as patellofemoral joint disease.

9. ++) Asking the athlete if he ever sustained a prior knee injury is an appropriate question during the history portion of the initial evaluation. (The athlete states he had a partial anterior cruciate tear of the right knee a year ago.)

10. +) Assessing the range of motion of the knee joint would be appropriate at this time. This demonstrates the athlete's willingness to move and assists in determining the level of disability. (The athlete has difficulty fully flexing and extending the knee.)

11. 0) Testing the strength of the athlete's hip abductors will not provide any information that will lead to determining the nature and extent of the knee injury.

12. 0) It is obvious from the opening scenario that this is a knee injury; having the athlete attempt toe raises would be unnecessary and inappropriate. (The athlete has difficulty doing this.)

13. ++) From the information given at the opening scenario and the mechanism of injury, performing a pivot shift test would be appropriate and should be performed bilaterally for comparison to the uninvolved extremity. (The test is inconclusive because the athlete is so guarded.)

Passing mark = 10 questions (correctly answered)

Section B

The current situation: The athlete is complaining of pain along the anteromedial joint line and medial retinaculum. The athlete felt a "pop" and has significant edema of the right knee. He has difficulty flexing and extending the knee and has a positive Lachman's test on the right knee.

Your immediate responsibility: Protect the knee from further injury and control the pain and swelling.

14. +) Issuing crutches with a toe-touch weightbearing status would be an appropriate action. (The athlete is more comfortable ambulating with crutches.)

15. ++) Applying ice and elevation of the injured extremity are appropriate actions during the initial phases of treatment. (The pain and swelling are controlled.)

16. ++) The team physician should be contacted to evaluate the athlete. (The team physician has training room hours that afternoon.)

17. 0) At this point, you realize this is not a patellofemoral joint problem. McConnell taping would be unnecessary and inappropriate. (The athlete questions why you are taping his kneecap.)

18. --) Applying heat to a swollen joint is contraindicated in the initial treatment of this injury. (The pain and swelling increase significantly.)

19. 0) Ordering a functional knee brace at this phase of treatment would be premature.

20. -) The application of pulsed ultrasound would be an inappropriate action. (The pain and swelling increase.)

Passing mark = 6 questions (correctly answered)

Section C

The current situation: The team physician has examined the athlete and agrees with your suspicions. The MRI results are pending.

Your immediate responsibility: Instruct the athlete in a home program emphasizing pain and edema reduction, early joint mobilization/range of motion, and isometric strengthening.

21. +) It is important to restore normal joint range of motion as soon as possible. This would be an appropriate action. (The athlete's range of motion improves 50% over the following week.)

22. ++) Applying ice on a routine basis during the initial stages of recovery is critical. (The pain and swelling decrease significantly.)

23. -) The athlete should remain on the crutches to protect the injured limb until the diagnosis is confirmed. (The athlete's knee buckles while walking with a cane and he falls.)

24. 0) Working on the proprioception of the unaffected limb is unnecessary. (The athlete's balance is fine.)

25. ++) Instructing the athlete to perform early isometric exercises is an appropriate step in preventing atrophy of the musculature around the knee joint. (The athlete is compliant.)

26. 0) The pain is controlled well with ice; a TENS unit is not contraindicated, but not necessary.

27. --) The athlete should be restricted from activities that may cause further injury until the diagnosis is confirmed and the athlete is cleared by the doctor. (The athlete re-injures his knee.)

Passing mark = 6 questions (correctly answered)

PROBLEM XI

Section A

The current situation: An athlete has requested assistance in developing a lower body strength and general conditioning program. He is currently in preseason.

Your immediate responsibility: Educate the athlete about the goals of preseason training and in proper methods to develop good habits to develop lower extremity flexibility strength. Assist the athlete in progressing his program and in preparing for his sport.

1. --) An athletic trainer is not qualified to administer steroids. This is an inappropriate action. (The athletic director finds out and you lose your job.)

2. +) A good flexibility program is a fundamental aspect of a general conditioning program. (The athlete's flexibility improves.)

3. --) Having the athlete participate in such a vigorous activity is inappropriate. (The athlete develops heat exhaustion.)

4. 0) There is nothing in the opening scene to indicate the athlete has a respiratory problem. This is an unnecessary action.

5. +) Adequate warm-up and cool-down periods are fundamental elements of a comprehensive fitness program. (The athlete had spent little time warming up prior to your recommendations.)

6. ++) Optimal results occur from training when the athlete mimics movement patterns and speeds that are similar to the activities he participates in (eg, training a soccer player by performing short, high intensity sprints).

7. -) Having the athlete participate in another sport such as tennis during the preseason may not be wise because of the increased risk of injury just before the season begins. (The athlete sprains his ankle and cannot participate for the first 2 weeks of the season.)

8. ++) Having the athlete work on the strength of his lower extremities would be appropriate.

9. -) The athlete should be assisted in maintaining a well-balanced nutritional diet. Limiting the athlete to one or two food groups is not appropriate. (The athlete complains of feeling lethargic.)

10. --) A regular training schedule should be maintained during the preseason period to allow for a progressive program. (Because of the many changes in the schedule during the preseason, the athlete is not in an acceptable state of fitness by the beginning of the season.)

11. --) Keeping the training schedule intense is acceptable, but often coaches prolong the workout, increasing the quantity rather than the quality of the session. (The athlete becomes overly fatigued and pulls a hamstring.)

12. ++) Progressing the conditioning program gradually is an appropriate action. (The athlete is at his physical peak going into the season.)

13. +) Making sure the athlete has acclimated to the heat prior to the season is appropriate. (The athlete avoids episodes of heat cramps or heat exhaustion.)

Passing mark = 10 questions (correctly answered)

Section B

The current situation: The athlete has started a preseason conditioning program as per your instructions to improve his lower body strength and general conditioning. He is now in-season.

Your immediate responsibility: Continue to supervise his program to maintain a proper level of fitness that is tailored for his sport and position, and add variety to prevent staleness.

14. +) Establishing a regular aerobic exercise routine while in-season is an appropriate action. (The athlete maintains a good aerobic conditioning level.)

15. ++) Maintaining a regular strength training program throughout the season is appropriate. (The athlete maintains a good strength level for his lower extremities.)

16. --) Rest is important, but too much time off while in-season is counterproductive. (The athlete starts to show signs of deconditioning.)

17. 0) This action is unnecessary unless the athlete has a known or suspected cardiovascular problem.

18. +) This is an appropriate action depending on the athlete's position. (The athlete is a running back.)

19. ++) Establishing a maintenance program for training while in season is necessary and appropriate. (The athlete maintains a good level of aerobic and strength conditioning.)

20. -) Putting the athlete on a clear diet is inappropriate. (The athlete begins to show signs of fatigue and malnutrition.)

21. +) Cross-training during the season may serve to maintain a good fitness level and prevent staleness during training. (The athlete swims one to two times per week.)

22. 0) Although this action is not harmful, it is not sport specific and is not a necessary activity.

23. --) This action is not necessary and is inappropriate. (The athlete is thrown during a competition and is injured.)

Passing mark = 8 questions (correctly answered)

Section C

The current situation: It is now postseason. The athlete has done well thus far with the conditioning program you have designed.

Your immediate responsibility: Continue to educate the athlete regarding proper flexibility and strengthening techniques. Adjust the workload so the athlete will avoid boredom and maintain a good level of fitness at a lower intensity.

24. ++) Maintaining a good flexibility program year-round is appropriate. (The athlete remains injury free during the off-season.)

25. ++) Cross-training is appropriate during the entire year but is especially effective during the off-season period to maintain proper fitness levels and prevent boredom with training. (The athlete uses a rowing machine during the off-season.)

26. --) The off-season is a period of detraining, where there is a gradual decrease of the workload. Jogging 4 to 5 days a week would be inappropriate. (The athlete shows signs of overtraining and quits the team.)

27. --) Along with a decrease in activity intensity during the off-season, there should be a decrease in the calorie intake by the athlete. Having the athlete consume a high-calorie diet during the off-season is inappropriate. (The athlete reports to preseason practice 10 pounds overweight.)

28. 0) Having the athlete learn the skill of visual imagery may enhance performance techniques but is not a necessary activity in maintaining fitness during the off-season.

29. --) Having the athlete become completely sedentary during the off-season period is inappropriate. (The athlete gains 20 pounds during this time and becomes aerobically unfit).

30. +) Allowing the athlete time off from training will prevent burnout. (The athlete appreciates the much-needed break.)

31. +) Participating in another sport during the off-season will help the athlete maintain a proper level of fitness. (The athlete plays basketball during the off-season.)

Passing mark = 6 questions (correctly answered)

Problem XII

Section A

The current situation: You know your athlete has suffered a serious traumatic injury after colliding with the boards.

Your immediate responsibility: To perform your initial evaluation to determine the nature and severity of the injury and assess if it is a life-threatening situation.

1. -) Performing a secondary survey prior to doing a primary survey would be premature and inappropriate. (The athlete is in respiratory distress and you have wasted valuable time.)

2. ++) If the athlete is lying prone and it has been determined he is not breathing, this would be an appropriate action. (The athlete is unconscious and not breathing.)

3. --) This is an inappropriate action. The helmet should not be removed until a neck or spinal injury has been ruled out. (The athlete has sustained a spinal cord injury and is now a quadriplegic.)

4. ++) Determining responsiveness and the ABCs is the immediate priority. This is an appropriate action. (The athlete is unconscious and not breathing.)

5. ++) This is an appropriate action. Determining level of consciousness is part of the primary survey.

6. --) Chest compressions should not be started unless it has been established that the athlete is pulseless. (The athlete has a weak carotid pulse.)

7. 0) This would be an inappropriate action. It is apparent from the opening scenario that the primary site of injury is not an extremity.

8. -) This is an unnecessary action. It is known from the opening scenario that the athlete hit the boards with his head. (You spend too much time asking questions instead of evaluating the athlete.)

9. --) This is an inappropriate action. The athlete should not be moved until a neck or back injury has been ruled out.

Passing mark = 7 questions (correctly answered)

Section B

The current situation: The athlete has been carefully placed into supine and is unconscious and not breathing. He has a weak pulse.

Your immediate responsibility: Establish an airway and ventilate the athlete. Activate the EMS system.

10. -) The immediate priority is establishing an airway. Performing a secondary survey is inappropriate at this time. (The athlete has now been without oxygen for 1.5 minutes.)

11. +) This would be an appropriate action, as a true emergency has been determined. (The ambulance arrives within 5 minutes of the call.)

12. --) This is an inappropriate action and may cause further injury to the athlete.

13. 0) Although this action is appropriate, it is not a priority at this time.

14. ++) Cutting the face mask off the helmet is a necessary step to allow for CPR and artificial respiration. (You are now able to ventilate the athlete.)

15. -) This is an unnecessary and inappropriate action.

16. -) This is an unnecessary and inappropriate action. (The Romberg sign is a test used to assess balance.)

17. --) This is an inappropriate action. (The athlete vomits, aspirates, and dies.)

18. ++) This is an appropriate action; opening the airway and ventilating the athlete is a priority. (You are able to open the airway and administer mouth-to-mouth respiration.)

19. 0) This action is unnecessary as it has already been determined the athlete has a pulse.

20. +) Removing the mouthguard is necessary to clear the airway. This is an appropriate action.

21. +) Using a jaw-thrust to open the airway is an appropriate action. (You suspect a possible spinal cord injury.)

Passing mark = 10 questions (correctly answered)

Section C

The current situation: The athlete responds to your resuscitation efforts and becomes conscious and is able to respond to questions. He reports feelings of gross anesthesia.

Your immediate responsibility: Assess and monitor the athlete's vital signs, assess the extent of loss of sensation and motor control, and document what occurred and who was involved. Prepare to transport the athlete to the hospital via ambulance.

22. ++) Once the athlete is conscious and breathing independently, it is a priority to perform a secondary survey. (Respiratory rate is 14 breaths per minute, blood pressure is 110/70, and pulse is 88. Gross sensation is absent from the armpits caudally, no significant bleeding or deformities noted.)

23. +) Monitoring the athlete's vital signs is appropriate. (You are able to give the EMS team vital information.)

24. -) This is an inappropriate action. (You do not have enough information regarding the athlete's permanent outcome.)

25. +) This is an appropriate action. (The athlete is ready to be transferred to the hospital.)

26. 0) This would be an inappropriate action at this time. (This would not be helpful at this time.)

27. +) Checking the pupillary response is an appropriate action to determine if the athlete has sustained a head injury. (Both pupils respond normally.)

28. -) This is an inappropriate action. (The policy on helmet removal should be established before a catastrophic injury occurs.)

29. -) This is an inappropriate action. Once the athlete is transferred into the care of the emergency medical team, you are still responsible for the remaining athletes. (You leave the practice area and a second athlete gets injured.)

30. +) This would be an appropriate action. (You avoid a malpractice suit.)

Passing mark = 7 questions (correctly answered)

Section D

The current situation: Your athlete has suffered a serious spinal cord injury and has been transported by the rescue squad to the hospital.

Your immediate responsibility: Provide emotional support to the athlete and his teammates. Provide accurate information of what occurred to the team physician and provide support for the athlete's parents.

31. ++) This would be an appropriate action. (The athlete is very scared and is grateful you came.)

32. +) This is an appropriate action. (The team doctor documents what occurred.)

33. +) This is an appropriate action. (The parents meet you at the emergency room.)

34. --) This is an inappropriate action. An athletic trainer is not qualified to determine the athlete's prognosis. (You have given the athlete false hope and he becomes severely depressed.)

35. 0) This is an unnecessary action. (It is too late to change this now.)

36. --) This is an inappropriate action. (You are reprimanded by the school administration.)

37. +) This is an appropriate action. (The coach appreciates the information.)

38. +) This is an appropriate action. (The rest of the hockey team express how they are feeling.)

39. -) This is an inappropriate action. (The physician never makes the phone call and the athletic director finds out about the accident the following day from a coach.)

Passing mark = 7 questions (correctly answered)

PROBLEM XIII

Section A

The current situation: An athlete comes to you complaining of right shoulder pain that occurs after throwing. He is able to voluntarily sublux both his shoulders.

Your immediate responsibility: To perform an initial evaluation to determine the nature and severity of the problem.

1. ++) Asking the athlete how long the problem has existed is a fundamental question to ask during the history portion of the evaluation. This will give the athletic trainer an idea if this is an acute or chronic problem. (The athlete states it has hurt over the past 3 weeks.)

2. +) A more appropriate question might be to ask the athlete if the right shoulder had ever been injured in the past and when the injury occurred. (The athlete states he has not had a shoulder injury prior to this recent episode.)

3. +) This is an appropriate question to ask during the history portion of the evaluation. (The athlete states that he cannot specifically tell you what position[s] make the pain worse.)

4. 0) This would be an inappropriate question. Whether or not the athlete is consuming an adequate amount of protein has nothing to do with this problem.

5. ++) This would be an appropriate question given the information that has been provided in the opening scenario. (The fact that the athlete is able to voluntarily sublux his shoulder.)

6. 0) This question is unnecessary and inappropriate. The athlete has already provided you with information in the opening scenario relating to his joint laxity.

7. 0) This question is unnecessary and inappropriate. Whether or not the athlete is taking supplemental vitamins has no direct correlation to the present problem.

8. +) Asking the athlete about the intensity of his pain will provide the athletic trainer information regarding the severity of the condition. (The athlete reports his pain level is moderate, 5/10 after pitching.)

9. -) This is an inappropriate question. Whether or not his father played baseball is irrelevant and whether or not his father had injured his shoulder has no direct correlation to the present problem. (The athlete has no idea if his father ever had a shoulder problem.)

10. +) Asking the athlete about any medications he may be taking is appropriate during the history portion of the initial evaluation. (The athlete reports he has been taking aspirin for the pain with temporary relief.)

Passing mark = 8 questions (correctly answered)

Section B

The current situation: The athlete has subacute right shoulder pain with joint laxity. He is able to voluntarily sublux both his shoulders. Aspirin provides minimal pain relief.

Your immediate responsibility: Perform special tests to identify the etiology of the athlete's pain.

11. -) This is an inappropriate test for this problem. The Phalen's test is performed when carpal tunnel syndrome is suspected.

12. +) A Clunk test is an appropriate test to perform if a glenoid labral tear is suspected. (The athlete has a negative Clunk test.)

13. -) The pivot shift test is performed to evaluate the knee for anterolateral instability secondary to tearing the anterior cruciate ligament. This is an inappropriate test for this problem.

14. -) The Patrick's test is performed to evaluate the hip for iliopsoas, sacroiliac, or joint pathology. This is an inappropriate test for this problem.

15. -) A Thompson test is performed when the possibility of an Achilles' tendon rupture exists. This is an inappropriate test for this problem.

16. +) The apprehension test (anterior and posterior) is an appropriate test to perform for this problem. A positive test may be indicative of either anterior or posterior glenohumeral instability. (The athlete has a positive apprehension sign.)

17. +) The Hawkin's-Kennedy impingement test is used to test for pain and apprehension relating to shoulder impingement. This would be an appropriate test to perform for this problem. (The athlete has a positive Hawkin's test.)

18. +) The Neer test is used to test for pain and apprehension relating to shoulder impingement, primarily of the biceps long head and supraspinatus tendons. (The athlete has a negative Neer sign.)

19. +) The posterior drawer test of the shoulder is used when there is suspicion of posterior instability of the glenohumeral joint. This would be an appropriate test for this problem. (The athlete has a negative posterior drawer sign.)

20. -) The Ober test is used to determine iliotibial band/tensor fasciae latae tightness of the lower extremity. This is an inappropriate test for this problem.

21. -) A Trendelenburg test is used to determine if there is weakness of the gluteus medius muscle. This is not an appropriate test for this problem.

22. +) Testing for a sulcus sign is appropriate when assessing the athlete for multidirectional instability of the shoulder. This is an appropriate test for this problem. (The athlete has a positive sulcus sign.)

Passing mark = 10 questions (correctly answered)

Section C

The current situation: The athlete has a positive impingement test, a positive sulcus sign, and a positive apprehension test.

Your immediate responsibility: Instruct and supervise an upper extremity strengthening program.

23. +) Shoulder shrugs strengthen the upper trapezius muscle, which helps to stabilize the scapula superiorly.

24. -) Although bicep curls are not inappropriate for general upper extremity strengthening, they will not contribute to strengthening the rotator cuff or scapula musculature.

25. +) Shoulder abduction strengthening exercises are appropriate, as they stabilize the scapula laterally and posteriorly.

26. -) Cervical isometric exercises are unnecessary and inappropriate for this particular problem, as they will not have a direct effect on stabilizing the scapula or strengthening the rotator cuff.

27. ++) Resistive exercises involving internal and external rotation of the shoulder directly strengthen the rotator cuff musculature.

28. +) Resistive exercises performed in the D2 extension pattern work the shoulder extensors, adductors, and internal rotators. This type of exercise would be appropriate for this problem.

29. -) Because the long head of the triceps brachii muscle arises from the infraglenoid tuberosity of the scapula, shoulder extension exercises would assist in scapular stabilization, but tricep curls (ie, elbow extension) would not have a direct effect on either the scapula or the rotator cuff.

30. +) Rowing exercises strengthen the rhomboids, triceps (long head) and latissimus dorsi, stabilizing the scapula medially and posteriorly.

31. +) Exercises involving resisted scapular protraction strengthen the serratus anterior muscle, stabilizing the scapula laterally.

32. -) Partial sit-ups strengthen the upper abdominals, which is unnecessary and inappropriate for this problem.

33. -) Prone trunk extensions strengthen the erector spinae musculature of the back, which is unnecessary and inappropriate for this problem.

34. -) Calf raises strengthen the triceps surae complex of the lower leg, which is unnecessary and inappropriate for this problem.

Passing mark = 10 questions (correctly answered)

PROBLEM XIV

Section A

The current situation: You know your athlete has sustained a left lower leg injury and the mechanism of injury was an indirect trauma.

Your immediate responsibility: To perform your initial evaluation of the injury to determine the type and extent of the injury.

1. -) It is obvious from the opening scenario that the athlete is breathing fine. (The athlete is howling in pain.)

2. -) It is obvious from the opening scenario that the athlete has a significant lower extremity injury; it is inappropriate to have the athlete attempt to walk until your initial evaluation is complete. (The athlete asks if you are a student trainer.)

3. +) Asking the athlete what happened is an appropriate question that should be asked during the history portion of the initial evaluation. (He states he stopped suddenly and the left lower leg "gave out.")

4. -) It is obvious from the opening scenario that the athlete has not sustained a head injury. This would be an inappropriate action. (The athlete is very alert and in severe pain.)

5. +) Examining the athlete's leg for areas of external or internal bleeding (ecchymosis) is an appropriate action. (There are no obvious signs of bleeding at this time.)

6. ++) Asking the athlete where the pain is located is fundamental in determining what structures of the lower leg are involved. (The athlete points to the musculotendious junction of the gastrocnemius and Achilles'.)

7. ++) Observing the area of injury is an appropriate and necessary action as part of the initial assessment of an injury. (There is mild edema of the posterior lower extremity at the musculotendious junction.)

8. ++) Asking the athlete whether or not he felt or heard a "pop" or "snap" provides the athletic trainer information regarding the nature and severity of the injury. (The athlete states he felt a "pop" with severe pain in the calf.)

9. 0) Applying ice at this point of your evaluation will not hurt the athlete but is premature, as your evaluation is not yet complete.

10. -) Asking the athlete if he has ever injured his uninvolved leg would be inappropriate at this time, as it is not a priority. (The athlete states his left lower extremity has never been hurt.)

11. --) It is obvious from the opening scenario that the left lower extremity has been significantly injured. Asking the athlete to stand and hop would be inappropriate and could cause further injury if attempted. (The athlete completely ruptures his gastrocnemius muscle.)

Passing mark = 9 questions (correctly answered)

Section B

The current situation: You know from your evaluation that the athlete felt a "pop" accompanied by severe pain at the musculotendinous junction of the gastrocnemius and Achilles' tendon. There is mild edema present in the area.

Your immediate responsibility: To continue your evaluation to determine the severity of the injury.

12. ++) Palpating the injured extremity for swelling and deformity would be an appropriate action at this time. (There is now a moderate effusion of the lower extremity and a palpable defect at the musculotendinous junction.)

13. -) Performing a Lachman's test bilaterally would be an unnecessary and inappropriate action. The injury is to the left lower extremity, not the knee. (The athlete wonders why you are checking his knee.)

14. -) Performing a Thomas test bilaterally would be an unnecessary and inappropriate action. The Thomas test is performed to assess for tight hip flexors. (You have now wasted time examining the athlete's hip flexibility.)

15. +) Checking the active range of motion of both ankles is appropriate to assess the athlete's functional ability and willingness to move. (The athlete is unable to actively plantar flex his foot and has pain with the attempt.)

16. -) Checking the athlete's Q-angle is unnecessary and inappropriate. It is also known from the opening scenario that is it the left lower extremity, not the right, that is injured. (Be sure to carefully read through all the information provided.)

17. 0) Whether or not the athlete has bunions has nothing to do with this injury.

18. ++) Performing a Thompson test bilaterally would be an appropriate action to take during your assessment of this injury. (The test is positive on the left leg.)

19. -) Performing a Hawkin's test bilaterally would be unnecessary and inappropriate. The athlete's right lower extremity has been injured, not his shoulder. (The athlete wonders why you are examining his shoulder.)

20. -) Performing an anterior drawer test bilaterally on both ankles is unnecessary and inappropriate. The athlete's left lower leg has been injured, not his left ankle. (The athlete wonders why you are examining his ankles.)

21. 0) Palpating the femoral pulse is unnecessary and inappropriate for this problem. (The athlete's femoral pulses are fine.)

22. 0) Testing the patellar tendon reflexes bilaterally is an unnecessary and inappropriate action. (The athlete's patellar tendon reflexes are fine.)

23. +) Testing the strength of the ankle plantar flexors would be an appropriate action to take when initially assessing the severity of the injury. (The strength of the ankle plantar flexors is -2/5 and painful.)

Passing mark = 10 questions (correctly answered)

Section C

The current situation: You suspect a torn left gastrocnemius muscle.

Your immediate responsibility: To begin treatment to control the pain and swelling and protect the athlete from further injury.

24. --) If the lower limb still has a significant amount of swelling, warm whirlpool treatments would be inappropriate. (The athlete's leg swells significantly during this treatment.)

25. ++) Applying ice to the injured area is an appropriate action to ease the pain and control the effusion. (The athlete is much more comfortable with the ice.)

26. ++) Applying a compression wrap to the injured area is an appropriate action to ease the pain and control the effusion. (The athlete is much more comfortable with the compression wrap.)

27. +) High-volt galvanic stimulation can be used to modulate pain and assist with edema reduction. (The athlete is much more comfortable after the treatment.)

28. ++) The application of a posterior leg splint is an appropriate action. This puts the lower extremity at rest and protects the area from further injury. (The athlete is much more comfortable with the lower leg immobilized.)

29. -) Attempting to use the Baps board too early in the treatment may increase pain and swelling. This is an inappropriate action at this time. (The athlete complains of increased calf pain and is frustrated he is unable to move the board.)

30. --) Based on your initial assessment, this athlete has sustained a torn gastrocnemius muscle. This would be an inappropriate action if your assessment is correct. (The athlete howls in pain during the attempt to come up on his toes.)

31. +) This is an appropriate action, especially if the lower extremity is immobilized.

32. -) This is an inappropriate action. The defect is a result of a torn muscle, not an infection. (The athlete questions why you are smearing gel on him.)

33. 0) The athlete may or may not be able to perform hamstring curls early in the rehabilitation. (The athlete is able to lift light weights.)

34. --) Because this is an acute muscle tear, ultrasound treatments are contraindicated at this time. (The calf swells and becomes ecchymotic.)

35. -) While gentle range of motion exercises are appropriate, the injured limb is the left lower extremity, not the right. (The athlete reminds you that his right leg is fine.)

Passing mark = 10 questions (correctly answered)

Section D

The current situation: Your athlete sustained a torn gastrocnemius muscle, which is now subacute in nature. The motion of his ankle and knee is normal, but he still has some strength deficits in plantar flexion.

Your immediate responsibility: Develop a strength and conditioning program designed to improve the athlete's left lower extremity strength and maintain his level of fitness.

36. ++) Stationary bicycling would be appropriate at this point of this athlete's rehabilitation. (The athlete is grateful to be aerobically active.)

37. --) Uphill jogging would be inappropriate. Based on the information provided, the athlete's strength in plantar flexion is still weak. This exercise is premature and may cause further injury. (The athlete retears the muscle.)

38. 0) Although push-ups will not harm the athlete, it is not a necessary exercise for this athlete's rehabilitation.

39. ++) Having the athlete performing progressive-resistive ankle exercises in all directions would be appropriate at this point of the athlete's rehabilitation. (The athlete has no pain or significant difficulty with resistive exercises.)

40. --) Knowing from the information given thus far that the athlete is weak in plantar flexion concentrically, plyometric exercises would be inappropriate and may cause further injury if initiated too soon. (The athlete retears the gastrocnemius.)

41. 0) Using the upper body ergometer during the athlete's rehabilitation would be appropriate to maintain aerobic fitness but is not directly related to rehabilitating a lower extremity injury.

42. +) Initiating exercises that enhance proprioception is a necessary and appropriate action to take in preparing the athlete to return to his sport. (The athlete demonstrates some difficulty in maintaining his balance on the injured leg.)

43. ++) Having the athlete perform exercises that directly work in strengthening the plantar flexors of the ankle is appropriate. (The athlete has no pain performing this exercise but still has difficulty performing unilateral calf raises.)

44. +) Partial squats with and without additional resistance is appropriate for lower extremity strengthening. (The athlete is able to do this without pain or difficulty.)

45. ++) Having the athlete perform resisted hamstring curls would be appropriate, as the gastrocnemius not only functions to plantar flex the ankle but is also a flexor of the knee.

46. +) It is important to make sure the rest of the leg is strengthened in addition to the specific area of injury, because the entire lower extremity loses strength during the initial phases treatment when the limb is immobilized. (The athlete has normal quadricep strength bilaterally.)

47. +) Making sure the athlete maintains his lower extremity flexibility is appropriate in preparing the athlete to return to his sport. (The athlete's flexibility is normal bilaterally.)

48. -) Focusing attention on upper extremity strengthening would not be necessary or appropriate during the rehabilitation of this injury.

49. -) Focusing attention on upper extremity strengthening would not be necessary or appropriate during the rehabilitation of this injury.

50. -) Until the strength of the athlete's plantar flexors on the injured limb is equal to the strength of the uninjured limb, initiating agility exercises would be inappropriate.

Passing mark = 12 questions (correctly answered)

Section E

The current situation: This athlete has been performing a general lower extremity flexibility and strengthening exercise program as instructed without complaints of pain or difficulty. He is anxious to return to playing competitive tennis.

Your immediate responsibility: Reassess the athlete and have the athlete perform a series of functional exercises to determine if the athlete is ready to play.

51. +) Making sure the athlete can walk without a limp would be appropriate. (The athlete has no difficulty with this task.)

52. ++) The athlete should be completely pain-free at rest and during activity prior to returning to full-time competition. (The athlete is completely pain-free.)

53. ++) There should be no visible edema or ecchymosis at the site of injury. (There is no visible swelling or ecchymosis.)

54. +) The athlete should have no complaints of pain with deep palpation of the injured area. (The athlete reports he has no pain with palpation of the injured area.)

55. +) The athlete should have no complaints of pain with a resisted hamstring curl. (The athlete is pain-free with this motion.)

56. ++) The athlete should have full range of motion of both the ankle and knee before returning to full activity. (The range of motion of the injured ankle and knee is equal to the uninjured side.)

57. --) The athletic trainer should only return the athlete to competition when the athletic trainer and team physician determine the athlete is fully recovered. (The athlete returns too soon and is re-injured.)

58. +) The athlete should be able to hop on the injured lower extremity without pain before returning to full activity. (The athlete has no pain or difficulty pushing off or landing on the injured leg.)

59. +) The athlete should be able to jog a reasonable amount of time in a straight line before returning to full activity. (The athlete has no difficulty doing this.)

60. --) Although the athlete may not be as interested in his rehabilitation program as he is in his sport, the athlete's level of interest is not a credible parameter by which to determine whether or not he can return to full activity.

61. ++) The strength of the athlete's involved ankle should be equal to the strength of the uninvolved ankle before returning the athlete to full activity. (Both ankles are now graded as 5/5 during manual muscle testing.)

62. ++) It is prudent to have the team physician clear the athlete for return to full activity before the athlete participates in his sport. (The athlete is cleared for competition.)

63. 0) Whether or not the athlete can bench press 50 pounds or more has nothing to do with whether or not this athlete can compete in tennis. (The athlete can bench press 90 pounds.)

Passing mark = 10 questions (correctly answered)

PROBLEM XV

Section A

The current situation: You know from this athlete's complaints that his low back pain is chronic in nature and localized to the lumbar area.

Your immediate responsibility: To perform an initial evaluation to determine the etiology of his pain.

1.   ++) When assessing a low back injury, it is appropriate to observe the athlete's posture in standing and sitting. (The athlete stands with a forward head and rounded shoulder posture and slouches when he sits. The athlete also has a slight scoliotic curve.)

2.   +) Having the athlete describe his pain is appropriate, as it gives the athletic trainer information about the nature of the injury. (The athlete reports the pain is a "dull ache.")

3.   0) Checking the range of motion of the athlete's knees would not contribute any helpful information. This athlete has a low back problem, not a knee injury.

4.   -) A Scour test of the hip is performed when the possibility of hip arthritis exists. This test would be unnecessary and inappropriate. The athlete is not complaining of any hip pain.

5.   ++) Palpating the lumbar erector spinae is an appropriate action and is a fundamental component of the initial assessment. (The athlete reports mild muscle discomfort.)

6.   +) Although it is not likely that muscular wasting will be observed, it is appropriate to visualize the area of injury for any unusual changes such as atrophy, swelling, or deformity. (There is no evidence of muscular atrophy.)

7.   +) Palpation of the entire lumbar and sacral regions is appropriate during the initial evaluation to check for any areas of point tenderness. (The athlete is pain-free with palpation of both PSIS and SI joints.)

8.   0) Genu varum is a "bow-legged" deformity of the lower extremities and has no correlation to the athlete's low back pain.

9.   ++) Assessing the athlete for a leg-length discrepancy is appropriate. Even a subtle leg-length discrepancy can cause chronic low back pain. (The athlete's legs are of equal length.)

10.   0) Having the athlete perform a partial squat is unnecessary and inappropriate during the initial evaluation. Whether or not the athlete can perform this action will not provide the athletic trainer with significant information concerning the nature of the problem.

11.   ++) Evaluating the range of motion of the lumbar spine will help the athletic trainer assess the athlete's willingness to move and provide information concerning the nature and severity of the problem. (The athlete complains of pain with lumbar flexion, right side-bending, and right rotation.)

12.   -) Evaluating the athlete's hip abduction with a goniometer is not appropriate. This athlete does not have a hip injury.

13.   +) It would be appropriate to check the flexibility of the muscles around the hip because tight hip flexors or hamstrings can contribute to chronic low back pain. (The athlete has tight hamstrings bilaterally.)

Passing mark = 10 questions (correctly answered)

Section B

The current situation: You have determined from your initial evaluation that the athlete's pain is muscular in origin and he has tight bilateral hamstrings.

Your immediate responsibility: To provide immediate pain relief during rest and activity.

14.   -) Friction massage is a deep, local massage technique which is most commonly performed around joints and over thin tissue areas that are hypomobile because of scarring or local spasms. This type of massage is inappropriate for this problem. (The athlete complains of significant pain during treatment.)

15. ++) The application of ice in the form of ice packs can break the pain-muscle spasm-pain cycle, allowing the athlete to move more comfortably and is an appropriate modality to use. (The athlete reports pain relief during treatment.)

16. +) Because the injury is chronic in nature, and the athlete is not in severe pain, moist heat in the form of a whirlpool may be useful in helping the athlete relax and will reduce discomfort. (The athlete reports pain relief with the heat treatments.)

17. ++) Because this is a chronic problem, ultrasound would be an appropriate modality choice. Deep heat improves circulation, which enhances healing.

18. -) Iontophoresis is a technique in which ions of a chemical substance are delivered through the skin through use of an electrical current. The most common application is the delivery of a steroid to reduce a local inflammatory response (eg, tendinitis). Iontophoresis would not be an appropriate modality choice for this problem. (The athlete complains of irritation under the active electrode.)

19. 0) Although an ice massage would not harm the athlete, it would not be the optimal choice for decreasing chronic, diffuse low back pain. The application of ice massage would be more appropriate for decreasing pain in areas of point tenderness. (The athlete is not pleased with you rubbing ice all over his lower back.)

20. -) Sending the athlete for chiropractic treatments would not be appropriate. It is within the athletic trainer's scope of practice to be able to comprehensively manage this athlete's problem. (The chiropractor sends you a thank you note.)

21. +) TENS therapy would be an appropriate choice of a modality in managing the athlete's pain. (The athlete reports pain relief when the unit is used.)

22. ++) The application of moist heat packs (especially prior to exercise) would be appropriate to enhance relaxation and reduce pain. (The athlete reports pain relief with moist heat treatments.)

23. +) Short-wave diathermy would be an appropriate modality choice for treatment of chronic low back pain. Short-wave diathermy is a deep heater, which improves local circulation and enhances healing. (The athlete reports feeling better after treatment.)

24. 0) Although stationary bicycling would be appropriate for aerobic conditioning, it has no direct effect regarding pain reduction of the low back or improving lumbar movement.

25. --) Functional electric stimulation is not an appropriate modality choice in the treatment of chronic low back pain. It is primarily used for neuromuscular re-education. (The athlete has more pain because of the muscular stimulation.)

26. --) Cervical traction would not be an appropriate modality for this problem. This athlete has a low back problem, not a neck injury. (Please read the opening scenario.)

27. --) Paraffin bath would not be an appropriate modality choice for this problem. Paraffin treatments are most commonly used for hand and foot conditions. (The athlete is very upset that you are pouring a very warm waxy substance on his back.)

28. ++) Effleurage would be an appropriate action to take. This massage technique can be very effective in relaxing the athlete and in encouraging improved venous and lymphatic drainage. (The athlete reports significant relief of his muscular discomfort after your treatment.)

29. +) A neoprene lumbar support would be an appropriate item to recommend to the athlete to use during activity. It provides warmth and a sense of support which is effective in reducing pain with movement. (The athlete reports he is able to move easier during practice.)

Passing mark = 13 questions (correctly answered)

Section C

The current situation: The athlete's low back pain is beginning to reduce with the treatment he has been receiving by the athletic trainer.

Your immediate responsibility: To instruct the athlete in a series of exercises to improve his lumbar mobility and strength.

30. -) Active trunk extensions against gravity would be inappropriate in the initial stages of rehabilitation, especially while the athlete still is complaining of lumbar pain with active movement. This may aggravate his lumbar pain. (The athlete is fine extending his back while standing but reports increased pain attempting this in prone.)

31. +) Gentle active-assisted low back flexibility exercises, such as knee to chest exercises, are useful in the initial phases of rehabilitation to restore lumbar movement. (The athlete has minimal discomfort with these exercises.)

32. 0) Resisted knee extensions will not cause further injury to the athlete but are not necessary in the initial treatment of chronic low back pain. (The athlete has strong hip flexors and quadriceps.)

33. ++) Stretching the hamstrings would be an appropriate action to take. Tight hamstrings can contribute to chronic low back pain. (The athlete has bilateral tight hamstrings.)

34. ++) Having the athlete perform active posterior pelvic tilts would be an appropriate exercise to initiate during the early phases of rehabilitation. (The athlete has no difficulty or pain with this exercise.)

35. +) Stretching the hip flexors would be appropriate if it is found during the initial evaluation that the muscles were tight. If the hip flexors are too tight, it can place a strain on the low back area. (The athlete's hip flexors flexibility is within normal limits bilaterally.)

36. +) Strengthening the muscles around the hip is important because these muscles also serve to support the pelvis and lumbar areas. This would be an appropriate exercise only if it does not cause the athlete further discomfort.

37. +) Lower trunk rotations in supine are useful in the initial phases of rehabilitation to restore lumbar movement. (The athlete has no discomfort with these exercises.)

Passing mark = 6 questions (correctly answered)

Section D

The current situation: The athlete now has no complaints of low back pain during rest or activity.

Your immediate responsibility: Progress the athlete's program with an emphasis on lumbar stabilization to prevent a reoccurrence of low back pain.

38. ++) PNF exercises for the trunk would be appropriate as long as the chosen exercises cause the athlete no discomfort. (The athlete fatigues easily.)

39. ++) Resistive abdominal strengthening would be appropriate exercises to initiate during the later stages of rehabilitation as long as the exercises cause the athlete no discomfort. (The athlete fatigues easily.)

40. 0) Resistive cervical strengthening would be unnecessary and inappropriate for this problem.

41. +) Resisted prone hip extension requires activation of the lumbar musculature. This would be an appropriate exercise to perform for lumbar stabilization. (The athlete has no discomfort with this but fatigues easily.)

42. -) Achilles' stretching exercises are unnecessary and not appropriate for this problem. (The athlete questions why stretching his calves is important.)

43. -) Groin stretching exercises are unnecessary and not appropriate for this problem. (The athlete's groin musculature is not tight.)

44. --) Shoulder press exercises are unnecessary and inappropriate during the rehabilitation of this problem. Loading the spine with overhead exercises could cause further harm. (The athlete complains this exercise bothers his back.)

45. 0) Jogging would be appropriate to maintain aerobic conditioning but would not be the optimal choice of exercise for an athlete with a low back injury. Swimming would be a safer choice if a pool is available. (The athlete complains of mild lumbar discomfort with this activity but is able to jog short distances.)

46. ++) Swimming would be the optimal exercise for aerobic conditioning. (The athlete has no lumbar discomfort while swimming.)

47. ++) Resisted bridging exercises are an effective exercise for lumbar stabilization and are an appropriate exercise choice. (The athlete has no pain with this exercise.)

48. ++) In the late stages of rehabilitation, trunk extensions against gravity are appropriate to strengthening the erector spinae. (The athlete now has no complaints of lumbar discomfort but continues to fatigue easily with this exercise.)

Passing mark = 9 questions (correctly answered)

Problem XVI

Section A

The current situation: This athlete is complaining of ear pain and itching; you suspect the athlete has an ear infection.

Your immediate responsibility: Protect the athlete's ear to prevent the infection from getting worse and refer the athlete to a physician for treatment.

1. --) Dispensing antibiotics is a medical task, not an athletic training task. It is illegal for an athletic trainer to dispense antibiotics. (You are brought up on charges for practicing medicine.)

2. -) Cleaning the athlete's ear with epinephrine is an inappropriate action. Inserting any foreign object into the ear canal should be avoided. Epinephrine is a vasoconstrictor and is an inappropriate chemical for the treatment of external otitis. (The athlete hollers in pain during your attempt to "clean" his ear.)

3. +) It is important that the athlete is referred to the team physician as soon as possible so the athlete can begin treatment. (The athlete is placed on antibiotics by the team doctor.)

4. -) Protecting the ear that has an ear infection is best accomplished by plugging it with lamb's wool that is soaked with lanolin. (The athlete complains that the gauze pad is "not doing anything" and he removes it.)

5. +) It is best to avoid having the infected ear exposed to cold wind. Wearing a hood or hat that covers the ears will help protect the ear and reduce pain. (The athlete is much more comfortable when wearing a hood outside.)

6. --) The use of a TENS unit would not be appropriate in this situation. (Even the athlete knows this is wrong!)

7. -) Because swimmer's ear is caused by an infection as a result of fluid trapped in the ear canal, the application of a moist heat pack would not be an appropriate action. (The infection gets worse.)

8. +) It is appropriate to allow the athlete to continue swimming as long as the athlete habitually dries the affected ear with a soft towel and uses ear drops containing a 3% boric acid and alcohol solution before and after swimming.

Passing mark = 6 questions (correctly answered)

Section B

The current situation: The athlete has begun treatment by a physician.

Your immediate responsibility: Instruct the athlete in methods to prevent the infection from getting worse.

9.   ++) Using ear plugs while swimming to protect the infected ear is appropriate to reduce the amount of water entering the ear canal.

10. 0) Having the athlete utilize a bathing cap may help decrease the amount of water entering the ear while swimming but may not be totally effective in doing so if ear plugs are not used.

11. -) If properly managed, the athlete should be able to return to swimming on a regular basis.

12. 0) Wearing goggles is unnecessary and inappropriate regarding treatment of this problem.

13. ++) Having the athlete refrain from inserting any foreign objects into the ears is appropriate in protecting the athlete from further injury or additional infection.

Passing mark = 4 questions (correctly answered)

PROBLEM XVII

Section A

The current situation: You know your athlete has sustained an indirect traumatic injury to his right knee. He is able to bear weight without assistance.

Your immediate responsibility: To perform your initial evaluation to determine the nature and severity of the injury.

1.   ++) Having the athlete locate the area of pain is appropriate during the initial assessment of the injury. It is important in determining the nature of the injury. (The athlete reports he has pain along the medial side of the right knee.)

2.   +) Observing for areas of swelling is appropriate during the initial assessment of the injury. (There is minimal edema noted along the medial side of the right knee.)

3.   0) Applying ice to the area prior to completing the initial exam is a premature action.

4.   0) Applying a knee immobilizer prior to completing the initial examination is a premature action.

5.   0) Issuing a cane to the athlete prior to completing the initial examination is a premature action. A cane may or may not be an appropriate assistive device for this injury.

6.   ++) Palpation of the knee joint and the surrounding structures is a fundamental task of the initial evaluation. (The athlete reports he has a small amount of pain with palpation of the anteromedial joint line.)

7.   -) Palpating the gluteus medius muscle is an inappropriate and unnecessary action. It is obvious from the opening scenario that this is a knee injury, not a hip injury. (The athlete asks you why you are palpating his hip.)

8.   -) Having the athlete perform multiple calf raises is not an appropriate action. It is known from the opening scenario that the athlete has pain in full weightbearing. (The athlete is unable to perform a calf raise because of knee pain and instability.)

9.   ++) Evaluating the range of motion of both knees is appropriate during your initial evaluation of the injury. It assists the athletic trainer in determining the severity of the injury and the athlete's willingness to move. (The athlete has significant difficulty bending and completely straightening his knee because of pain.)

10. ++) Asking the athlete if he has injured his right knee before is an appropriate question during the history portion of the initial evaluation. (The athlete reports he had a minor knee injury 3 years ago but has been fine since that time.)

11. +) It is appropriate during the initial evaluation to assess the strength of the hip musculature bilaterally. (The strength of the hip flexors on the injured limb is 4+/5.)

12. +) It is appropriate during the initial evaluation to assess the strength of the quadriceps musculature bilaterally. (The strength of the quadriceps musculature on the injured limb is -3/5.)

13. +) It is appropriate during the initial evaluation to assess the strength of the hamstring musculature bilaterally. (The strength of the hamstring musculature on the injured limb is -3/5.)

14. 0) Checking the athlete's pupillary reaction is an unnecessary and inappropriate action. (The athlete tells you to get the light out of his eyes.)

Passing mark = 11 questions (correctly answered)

Section B

The current situation: You have determined from your evaluation that the athlete has pain along the medial aspect of the knee with palpation, there is minimal edema present, and the athlete has pain with movement into knee flexion and extension.

Your immediate responsibility: To continue your evaluation by performing special tests on the right knee.

15. ++) Performing a Lachman's test bilaterally would be appropriate to assess the integrity of the anterior cruciate ligament. (The Lachman's test is negative.)

16. --) The vertebral artery test is performed to test the patency of the vertebral arteries. This would be inappropriate. (The athlete does not trust you at this point of the exam.)

17. --) The Tinel's test is performed when carpal tunnel syndrome is suspected. This would not be an appropriate test for this problem. (The athlete reminds you that it is his knee that is injured, not his wrist or hand.)

18. ++) The valgus stress test is performed to test the integrity of the medial collateral ligament. Performing this test bilaterally would be appropriate. (The athlete complains of medial knee joint pain and there is increased valgus movement on the injured side.)

19. ++) The varus stress test is performed to test the integrity of the lateral collateral ligament. Performing this test bilaterally would be an appropriate action. (There is no complaint of pain with this test and minimal/no varus movement on the injured knee joint.)

20. +) Performing a posterior drawer test bilaterally would be appropriate to test the integrity of the posterior cruciate ligament. (The posterior drawer test is negative.)

21. --) The empty can test is performed to assess for supraspinatus weakness and is an inappropriate test for this problem. This athlete has a knee injury, not a shoulder injury. (The athlete's shoulders are fine.)

22. --) The Finkelstein test is performed to assess for tenosynovitis of the abductor pollicis longus and extensor pollicis brevis tendons and is an inappropriate test for this problem. (The athlete asks you what this test has to do with his knees.)

23. -) The Yergason's test is performed bilaterally when bicipital tendinitis is suspected. (The athlete asks you what this test has to do with his knees.)

24. ++) Performing a McMurray's test bilaterally would be appropriate to test the knee for a meniscal tear. (The McMurray's test is inconclusive because of the limitation in range of motion.)

25. +) Performing an anterior drawer test bilaterally would be appropriate to test the knee for an anterior cruciate tear. (The anterior drawer test is negative.)

26. +) Performing a pivot shift test would be appropriate to test the knee for anterolateral rotary instability secondary to a torn anterior cruciate ligament and posterolateral capsule. (The pivot shift test is inconclusive because the athlete is guarding.)

27. +) Performing a patellar apprehension test bilaterally would be appropriate to test the knee for patellar subluxation or dislocation. (The patellar apprehension test is negative.)

Passing mark = 10 questions (correctly answered)

Section C

The current situation: You suspect from the results of your evaluation that this athlete has a medial collateral ligament sprain with a possible meniscus tear of the right knee.

Your immediate responsibility: Begin a treatment program with emphasis on pain control and early motion.

28. --) The application of heat early in the rehabilitation when the knee is swollen would be inappropriate. (The knee swells severely after the heat is applied.)

29. -) Massaging the knee joint is unnecessary and inappropriate. (This causes great pain to the athlete and he avoids you the following week.)

30. --) Having the athlete attempt to use a rowing machine would be inappropriate during the initial stages of rehabilitation. (The athlete has significant knee pain and is unable to move the knee enough to operate it.)

31. ++) Placing the athlete on crutches to protect the joint is an appropriate action during the initial phases of treatment. (The athlete is much more comfortable and mobile with crutches.)

32. +) Assessing the strength of the quadriceps is important in determining the starting point for a rehabilitation program. (The athlete is unable to fully extend his knee against gravity.)

33. -) Starting isotonic hamstring strengthening exercises would be an inappropriate action if the goal is to treat the athlete for pain and swelling. (The athlete is unable to fully flex his knee against gravity.)

34. ++) Applying ice to the injured joint is appropriate for pain management and reducing edema. (The athlete reports pain relief with the ice packs in place.)

35. ++) It is important to have the athlete move his knee as soon as possible to his tolerance to maintain joint mobility. (The athlete is able to actively flex and extend his leg to a limited degree while lying in a supine position.)

36. 0) This would not be an appropriate suggestion. It is the right knee that has sustained the injury, not the left knee. (Make sure you read through the scenario carefully.)

37. --) It is not within an athletic trainer's scope of practice to issue medication with codeine as an active ingredient. (You are sued for trying to practice medicine.)

38. ++) The use of high-volt galvanic stimulation is indicated for reducing pain and swelling. (The athlete has good results with this treatment.)

Passing mark = 9 questions (correctly answered)

Section D

The current situation: The athlete's pain is controlled well with modalities and is moving his knee with greater ease.

Your immediate responsibility: To begin the athlete on a rehabilitation program with an emphasis on maintaining the athlete's aerobic conditioning and beginning functional exercises.

39. +) Functional activities should be introduced into the rehabilitation program as soon as possible; swimming is an appropriate activity to increase aerobic conditioning. (The athlete is able to swim with minimal discomfort.)

40. +) Having the athlete perform calf raises is an inappropriate activity as an early functional exercise.

41. -) Having the athlete attempt to run on a treadmill 1 week after sustaining a second-degree medial collateral tear of the knee would be inappropriate and may subject the athlete to further injury. (The athlete re-injures his knee while trying to run.)

42. +) Introducing closed-chain exercises such as stair-climbing (eg, Stairmaster) into the rehabilitation program as early as possible is an appropriate action. (The athlete is able to perform stair-climbing activities.)

43. ++) Having the athlete use the upper body ergometer to maintain aerobic fitness is appropriate. (The athlete is able to get a vigorous workout on this machine.)

44. 0) Wall pulley exercises for the upper extremity will not harm the athlete but are unnecessary and inappropriate if the goal is to maintain the athlete's aerobic capability.

45. ++) Introducing closed-chain exercises, such as stationary bicycling, into the rehabilitation program as early as possible is appropriate. (The athlete has minimal/no difficulty using the stationary bike.)

46. --) Fartlek training involves a type of cross-country running, which is varied in speed and terrain. This would be an inappropriate activity for the athlete to attempt early in the rehabilitation. (The athlete is unable to run, much less perform long-distance running through varied terrain.)

47. --) Plyometric exercises would be inappropriate in the early stages of rehabilitation. (The athlete attempts to jump up onto a stool from the floor and re-injures his knee.)

48. --) Resisted rowing early in the rehabilitation would be inappropriate. The ballistic motion may cause further pain or injury. (The athlete complains of significant pain during this activity.)

Passing mark = 8 questions (correctly answered)

PROBLEM XVIII

Section A

The current situation: You know this athlete has sustained a significant abdominal injury after being kicked by an opponent.

Your immediate responsibility: To perform an initial evaluation to determine the nature and extent of the injury and assess if it is a life-threatening situation.

1. ++) Performing a primary survey would be an appropriate action. (The athlete is conscious, coherent, and in obvious pain.)

2. 0) Giving the athlete oxygen is unnecessary and inappropriate. (The athlete angrily pushes the oxygen mask away from his face.)

3. -) Auscultating the athlete's heart is an inappropriate and unnecessary action. (The athlete's heart is fine.)

4. ++) It is appropriate to gently palpate the athlete's abdomen to assess for areas of pain and firmness. (The athlete has significant pain with palpation of the lower right quadrant and a moderately sized hematoma over the injury site.)

5. ++) It is appropriate during the history portion of the initial assessment to ask the athlete where the pain is located. This will give the athletic trainer an idea regarding the nature of the injury. (The athlete reports his pain is located in the lower right quadrant of his abdominal area.)

6. --) Having the athlete attempt to stand and jog in a premature action. You have not yet completed your evaluation and may cause further injury by excessively moving the athlete. (This athlete cannot stand, much less jog, because of the pain.)

7. 0) Having the athlete count backward from 100 would be inappropriate and unnecessary. It is known from the opening scenario that a head injury has not been sustained.

8. 0) Having a stretcher brought out to the field is a premature action, as the initial evaluation has not been completed.

9. 0) Unless there is any evidence of bleeding, donning latex gloves is not necessary.

10. ++) Observing the abdominal area for signs of edema or ecchymosis is fundamental during the initial assessment of the injury. (There is a contusion over the lower right quadrant.)

11. ++) Asking the athlete whether the pain radiates anywhere is essential in determining if there are any possible internal injuries and assessing the severity of the injury. (The pain is local to the area of injury.)

Passing mark = 9 questions (correctly answered)

Section B

The current situation: Your evaluation reveals a localized injury to the athlete's lower right abdominal area. The injury is not life-threatening.

Your immediate responsibility: Monitor the athlete's vital signs as a precaution. Begin treatment to control pain and minimize effusion.

12. ++) Applying an ice pack to the injured area would be appropriate to minimize pain and local effusion. (The athlete is much more comfortable with the ice treatment.)

13. +) Applying a compression wrap as soon as possible after the injury is appropriate to minimize pain and local effusion. (The athlete reports he feels a little better with the compression wrap in place.)

14. -) Massaging the athlete's lumbar area would be unnecessary and inappropriate. (The athlete questions what "rubbing his back" will do for him.)

15. --) Massaging the contused area will be irritating and encourage further bleeding into the area. (The athlete winces in pain.)

16. +) It would be appropriate to assist the athlete off the field so he can be monitored. (The athlete is able to walk off the field unassisted.)

17. 0) The application of a rib belt would be inappropriate for this injury.

18. +) It is appropriate to place the athlete in a position he is most comfortable, preferably in a position in which he is not placing pressure on the abdominals.

19. ++) It is important to monitor the athlete for any changes in pain location or intensity. This will alert the athletic trainer to any deterioration in the athlete's condition. (The athlete has no increase in pain 30 minutes after the injury.)

20. ++) Because of the possibility of internal injury, it is prudent to monitor the athlete's vital signs including his pulse and blood pressure. (The athlete's vital signs remain stable 1 hour after the incident.)

Passing mark = 7 questions (correctly answered)

Section C

The current situation: You have determined the athlete has sustained a moderate contusion to his lower right abdominal area. The pain and effusion has been well-controlled with your initial treatment.

Your immediate responsibility: Continue to use modalities to control the pain, monitor any changes in the athlete's condition, and protect the athlete from further injury.

21. ++) As long as the athlete has any pain, swelling, or ecchymosis present, it is appropriate to continue to apply ice to the injured area. (The athlete reports his pain is much less with the ice pack applied.)

22. -) Because the athlete is still complaining of pain, the application of moist heat packs would not be appropriate. (The athlete has some increased pain and swelling over the area of injury after treatment.)

23. --) A contusion to the abdominals is very painful and disabling to the athlete. Manually muscle testing the abdominals during the early phases of treatment is inappropriate. (The athlete has a difficult time rising from a supine position secondary to abdominal pain.)

24. +) It would be appropriate to re-evaluate the injury in greater depth the next day when the athlete is not in acute pain and there is more time to do so. (Your findings generally remain the same.)

25. 0) Although it is always important to keep an athlete well-hydrated, drinking a glass of Gatorade will not have any significant impact on the recovery of this athlete. (The athlete states he is not thirsty, but thanks you for your offer.)

26. ++) Protecting the injured area from further harm is appropriate and will give the athlete a sense of security. (The athlete is less apprehensive with the pad in place.)

27. +) Because this can be an incapacitating injury, maintaining the athlete's aerobic conditioning is critical during his recovery. Utilizing an upper body ergometer would be appropriate as long as the activity does not cause any discomfort. (The athlete has no difficulty with this activity.)

Passing mark = 6 questions (correctly answered)

Problem XIX

Section A

The current situation: You know this athlete has suffered a traumatic mouth/facial injury resulting from a blow by a hockey stick.

Your immediate responsibility: To perform an initial evaluation to determine the type and extent of the injury.

1. ++) Having the athlete clear the mouth with water and cleansing the face with water will allow the athletic trainer better visualization of the injured area.

2. -) Cleaning the athlete's mouth out with a paper towel is inappropriate. (The athlete is not pleased with pieces of paper sticking to her teeth and the roof of her mouth.)

3. ++) Anytime there is blood present during an injury, universal precautions must be observed.

4. -) The athlete has just received a significant blow to the mouth; wouldn't you be crying? (The athlete is upset with your insensitivity.)

5. +) It would be appropriate to check to see if the athlete was wearing a mouthguard. If she was wearing it, the fit must be checked. (She states she forgot it today and was not wearing it.)

6. -) Reviewing the school's liability insurance policy would be inappropriate. (It does not matter at this time.)

7. +) It would be an appropriate action to observe the mouth and surrounding areas for lacerations or abrasions. (There is an abrasion on the inside of the upper lip.)

8. +) Palpating the mouth and surrounding structures for deformity would be appropriate to check the athlete for a possible facial or jaw fracture. (Although edema is present, no gross deformity is palpable.)

9. -) Placing the athlete in a cervical collar would be unnecessary and inappropriate.

10. +) Having the athlete open and close her mouth will provide the athletic trainer some information concerning the extent of the injury. (The athlete is able to open and close her mouth, although it is painful.)

Passing mark = 8 questions (correctly answered)

Section B

The current situation: Your findings indicate that the athlete's inner upper lip has been abrased and there is some swelling present with a moderate amount of bleeding. There is no gross deformity of the face/jaw and the athlete is able to open and close her mouth. One of the athlete's front teeth is missing.

Your immediate responsibility: Recover the tooth, if possible, and try to reposition it, if possible. Refer the athlete to a dentist as soon as possible.

11. -) Asking the officials to stop the game would be unnecessary and inappropriate. (The officials deny your request.)

12. 0) Having a student trainer bring the athlete to the school nurse would be unnecessary and inappropriate. (There is nothing the school nurse could do that you could not do.)

13. +) Speaking with the athlete's parents would be appropriate, especially since the athlete is a minor. (The parents are grateful you filled them in on the situation.)

14. -) Calling the team physician would not be appropriate. (He wonders why you need his assistance.)

15. +) Applying ice to the injured area would be appropriate to control the athlete's pain and reduce the bleeding. (Although the athlete still has pain, she is more comfortable.)

16. +) Applying a cotton plug between the lip and injured gum will help control the bleeding and decrease the swelling. (The bleeding begins to stop.)

17. ++) Placing the displaced tooth in a container of sterile saline solution would be appropriate and is an important step toward saving the tooth if it is not possible to reposition the tooth in its socket.

18. +) The displaced tooth should be rinsed off with water to clean it of any dirt or debris.

19. ++) Sending the athlete and the tooth to a dentist within 30 minutes is critical if the tooth is to be saved. (The parents immediately leave with the athlete.)

20. --) Discarding the tooth is inappropriate unless it is a known fact that the tooth is no longer alive. (The parents threaten to sue you when they find out the tooth could have been saved.)

21. 0) Having the athlete lie down in a sidelying position has no bearing on this situation.

Passing mark = 9 questions (correctly answered)

PROBLEM XX

Section A

The current situation: You have been asked by an athlete to assist him in losing weight during his off-season period.

Your immediate responsibility: Assist the athlete in developing a nutritionally balanced diet and proper eating habits. Assess the athlete's current condition.

1. --) Having the athlete consume a protein drink daily with one of his regular meals will not encourage weight loss and should not be used in lieu of a regular meal. (The athlete gains another 7 pounds in 2 weeks.)

2. +) Using calipers to measure the athlete's percent body fat would be appropriate to obtain a baseline measurement. (The athlete's body fat is 12%.)

3. --) It is unrealistic to give the athlete a cookbook and expect him to lose weight as a result of that one action. This would be an inappropriate action. (The athlete admits he never even opened the book.)

4. --) Sending the athlete to an acupuncturist for this problem is not appropriate. (The athlete refuses to go.)

5. ++) Having the athlete record his food and drink intake in a personal log will assist the athletic trainer in adjusting the athlete's diet to ensure he is eating a nutritionally sound diet. (The athlete's current diet is high in fatty food and fluids high in sugar.)

6. ++) Monitoring the athlete's weight once a week will help the athletic trainer modify the athlete's diet accordingly and ensure the athlete is losing weight at a safe pace. (The athlete begins to lose weight after 3 days from initiating the new diet.)

7. --) Having the athlete fast is an inappropriate and potentially dangerous action. Fluids in particular should not be restricted. (The athlete becomes significantly dehydrated and ends up at the hospital.)

8. +) It is important that the athlete consume plenty of water while losing weight to avoid dehydration. (The athlete is compliant with this recommendation.)

9. ++) Weighing the athlete prior to beginning his program will provide the athletic trainer with a baseline weight, so weight reduction can be tracked. (The athlete is overweight by 10 pounds.)

10. --) Having the athlete sit in a sauna is an inappropriate and potentially dangerous suggestion. (The athlete sits in a sauna for an extended period of time and becomes significantly dehydrated.)

11. ++) Monitoring the athlete's exercise program is essential in providing a comprehensive weight loss program.

12. ++) Sitting down with the athlete to put together a balanced diet that he will adhere to is appropriate. Having the athlete be an active participant in his own care will help to maintain compliance. (The athlete is satisfied with the diet that is developed.)

13. --) Wearing a rubber suit during activity to encourage rapid dehydration is an inappropriate and very dangerous practice. (The athlete becomes severely dehydrated during a workout and collapses.)

14. 0) Although having the athlete perform progressive-resistive exercises for his lower extremities certainly will cause no harm to the athlete, it will serve no specific purpose in decreasing this athlete's weight. (In fact, the athlete's weight might increase with the increased muscle bulk.)

Passing mark = 11 questions (correctly answered)

Section B

The current situation: You have concluded from your assessment of this athlete that he is somewhat overweight and is eating a diet that is high in fat and sugar. He is compliant with your program and is beginning to show signs of success.

Your immediate responsibility: Continue to encourage the athlete in maintaining good eating habits and monitor the athlete on a regular basis to track his progression.

15. +) It would be appropriate to have the athlete keep a diet log so he can continue to keep track of what he eats and drinks. This will make it easier to make adjustments in his diet as necessary. (The athlete thinks this is a good idea.)

16. -) Having the coach monitor the athlete's food intake is inappropriate and not practical. (The coach has enough to do just coaching the team.)

17. ++) Having the athlete maintain a good level of hydration is always important. (This poses no problem.)

18. -) Increasing the level of physical activity does not necessarily require the athlete to exercise twice as long as his current exercise program requires. How the intensity and duration of the exercise program is modified will depend on the athlete's current level of activity. (The athlete becomes chronically fatigued.)

19. --) The use of laxatives to lose weight is inappropriate and potentially dangerous because of their dehydrating effects. (The athlete overdoses and collapses from dehydration and an electrolyte imbalance.)

20. 0) Involving a sports nutritionist is not necessary unless complicating conditions exist, such as medical problems (eg, diabetes, ulcerative colitis, etc) or the athlete desires to seek help from a professional nutritionist.

21. ++) To discourage binge eating, encouraging the athlete to eat numerous small meals throughout the day would be an appropriate suggestion. (The athlete nibbles on fruit, crackers, and small amounts of cheese during the day.)

22. 0) Although having the athlete perform progressive-resistive exercises for his upper extremities will cause him no harm, it serves no specific purpose in decreasing this athlete's weight. (The athlete sees no change in his weight since beginning an upper extremity strength program.)

Passing mark = 6 questions (correctly answered)

American Academy of Orthopedic Surgeons. *Athletic Training and Sports Medicine*. 2nd ed. Chicago, Ill: 1991.

Arnheim DD, Prentice WE. *Principles of Athletic Training*. 9th ed. St. Louis, Mo: Mosby Year Book Inc; 1997.

Cartwright, L. *Preparing for the Athletic Trainer's Certification Examination*. Champaign, Ill: Human Kinetics; 1995.

Crouch JE. *Functional Human Anatomy*. 4th ed. Philadelphia, Pa: Lea and Febiger; 1985.

DeVries HA. *Physiology of Exercise*. Dubuque, Iowa: Wm. C. Brown Co; 1980.

Fox S. *Human Physiology*. Dubuque, Iowa: Wm. C. Brown Co; 1984.

Gall MD, Gall JP, Jacobsen DR, Bullock TL. *Tools for Learning: A Guide to Teaching Study Skills*. Alexandria, Va: Association for Supervision and Curriculum Development; 1990.

Henry ML, Stapleton ER. *EMT Prehospital Care*. Philadelphia, Pa: WB Saunders Co; 1992.

Hollinshead WH. *Textbook of Anatomy*. 3rd ed. Philadelphia, Pa: Harper and Row Publishers; 1974.

Hoppenfeld S. *Physical Examination of the Spine and Extremities*. Norwalk, Conn: Appleton & Lange; 1976.

Hoppenfeld S, Zeide MS. *Orthopaedic Dictionary*. Philadelphia, Pa: JB Lippincott; 1994.

Kisner C, Colby LA. *Therapeutic Exercise: Foundations and Techniques*. 2nd ed. Philadelphia, Pa: FA Davis; 1991.

Konin JG. *Clinical Athletic Training*. Thorofare, NJ: SLACK Incorporated; 1997.

Konin JG, Wiksten DL, Isear J. *Special Tests for Orthopedic Examination*. Thorofare, NJ: SLACK Incorporated; 1997.

Kulund D. *The Injured Athlete*. Philadelphia, Pa: JB Lippincott; 1988.

Lehmkuhl LD, Smith LK. *Clinical Kinesiology*. 4th ed. Philadelphia, Pa: FA Davis Co; 1983.

Magee DJ. *Orthopaedic Physical Assessment*. Philadelphia, Pa: WB Saunders Co; 1992.

McFarlane P, Hodson S. *Studying Effectively and Efficiently: An Integrated System*. Toronto, Ontario, Canada: Governing Council of University of Toronto; 1983.

McMinn RMH, Hutchings RT. *A Colour Atlas of Human Anatomy*. London, England: Wolfe Medical Publications Ltd; 1998.

Mellion MB. *Sports Medicine Secrets*. Philadelphia, Pa: Hanley and Belfus Inc; 1993.

Mellion MB, Walsh WM, Shelton GL. *The Team Physician's Handbook*. Philadelphia, Pa: Hanley and Belfus Inc; 1990.

Michlovitz SL. *Thermal Agents in Rehabilitation*. 2nd ed. Philadelphia, Pa: FA Davis; 1990.

NATABOC. *Certification Update*. Dallas, Tex: NATA; 1999, Winter.

NATABOC. *Role delineation validation study for the entry level athletic trainers certification examination* (4th Ed.). Raleigh, NC: Columbia Assessment Services; 1999.

NATABOC. *Study Guide for the Entry-Level Athletic Trainer Certification Examination*. 2nd ed. Philadelphia, Pa: FA Davis Co; 1993.

Norkin C, Levangie P. *Joint Structure and Function. A Comprehensive Analysis*. 2nd ed. Philadelphia, Pa: FA Davis Co; 1992.

Norkin CC, White DJ. *Measurement of Joint Motion*. 2nd ed. Philadelphia, Pa: FA Davis Co; 1995.

Prentice WE. *Therapeutic Modalities in Sports Medicine*. 3rd ed. St. Louis, Mo: Mosby-Year Book Inc; 1994.

Ray R. *Management Strategies in Athletic Training*. Champaign, Ill: Human Kinetics Publishers; 1994.

Rothstein JM, Roy SH, Wolf SL. *The Rehabilitation Specialist's Handbook*. Philadelphia, Pa: FA Davis Co; 1991.

Roy S, Irvin R. *Sports Medicine: Prevention, Evaluation, Management and Rehabilitation*. Englewood Cliffs, NJ: Prentice-Hall Inc; 1983.

Sladyk K, McGeary S, Sladyk L, Tufano R. *OTR Exam Review Manual*. Thorofare, NJ: SLACK Incorporated; 1995.

Snyder-Mackler L. and Robinson AJ. *Clinical Electrophysiology: Electrotherapy and Electrophysiologic Testing*. Baltimore, Md: Williams and Wilkins; 1989.

Stedman's Medical Dictionary. 26th ed. Baltimore, Md: Williams & Wilkins; 1995.

Voss DE, Ionta MK, Myers BJ. *Proprioceptive Neuromuscular Facilitation*. 3rd ed. Phildadelphia, Pa: Harper and Row; 1985.

Wardlaw GM, Insel PM. *Perspectives in Nutrition*. 2nd ed. St. Louis, Mo: Mosby-Year Book Inc; 1993.

www.collegeboard.org/sat/html/tentips.html.

www.kdu.edu.my/tips.html.

www.lib2clark.cc.oh.us/library/studyhow.html.

www. nata.org.

www.NATABOC.org.

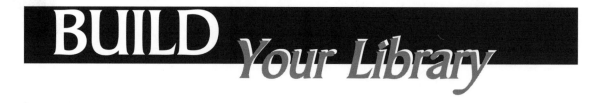
BUILD *Your Library*

This book and many others on numerous different topics are available from SLACK Incorporated. For further information or a copy of our latest catalog, contact us at:

Professional Book Division
SLACK Incorporated
6900 Grove Road
Thorofare, NJ 08086 USA
Telephone: 1-856-848-1000
1-800-257-8290
Fax: 1-856-853-5991
E-mail: orders@slackinc.com
www.slackbooks.com

We accept most major credit cards and checks or money orders in US dollars drawn on a US bank. Most orders are shipped within 72 hours.

Contact us for information on recent releases, forthcoming titles, and bestsellers. If you have a comment about this title or see a need for a new book, direct your correspondence to the Editorial Director at the above address.

Thank you for your interest and we hope you found this work beneficial.